The Headache
Prevention Cookbook

The Headache Prevention Cookbook

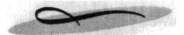

Eating Right to Prevent Migraines and Other Headaches

David R. Marks, M.D.

WITH

Laura Marks, M.D.

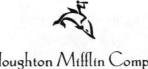

Houghton Mifflin Company
Boston   New York

For information about permission to reproduce selections from this book, write
to Permissions, Houghton Mifflin Company, 215 Park Avenue South,
New York, New York 10003.

Visit our Web site: www.hmco.com/trade.

Library of Congress Cataloging-in-Publication Data

Marks, David R.
The headache prevention cookbook : eating right to prevent migraines and other
headaches / David R. Marks, with Laura Marks.
p. cm.
Includes index.
ISBN 0-395-96716-3
ISBN 978-0-395-96716-4
1. Headache — Diet therapy — Recipes. 2. Headache — Prevention. I. Marks,
Laura. II. Title.

RC392 .M296 2000
616.8'4910654 — dc21   00-033435

Designed by Eugenie S. Delaney

Printed in the United States of America

DOH 10 9 8 7 6 5

This book is dedicated to our parents,
Lynne and Ralph Drabkin and Mimi and Stuart Marks.
We would never have made it here without you.
Sorry for any headaches we may have caused over the years.

Acknowledgments

RITING A BOOK is an enormous undertaking—more so than I ever imagined. Laura and I would never have finished if we hadn't received help from many people along the way.

I would like to thank Dr. Alan Rapoport and Dr. Fred Sheftell, cofounders and directors of the New England Center for Headache, who taught me virtually everything I know about the diagnosis and treatment of headaches. I would also like to thank the countless patients I have seen over the years. Their stories have been both heartbreaking and inspirational. There are few things more rewarding than helping a person avoid the misery of a headache.

A cookbook is only as good as its recipes. The following people deserve special thanks for contributing their own recipes: Lynne Drabkin, Julie Eckhert, Lauren Groveman, Julie Luchs, Michelle Cirino, Michele Cohen, Carol Bronz, Priscilla Alden van Cott, Mimi Marks, and my late grandmother, Rebecca Hanin.

I would like to thank Barry Estabrook, Lori Galvin-Frost, and the rest of the crew at Houghton Mifflin for their help in bringing this book to fruition.

I also owe a big thanks to my children, Jacob and Becca, for putting up with my crazy work schedule. You two are my biggest inspiration.

Thank you to my father-in-law, Ralph Drabkin, for all those days and nights you spent in Connecticut watching the kids while Laura and Mom cooked and I used the computer.

Finally, this book would have been impossible without the undying labor, devotion, and perseverance of four people:

Rux Martin, my editor at Houghton Mifflin, whose vision, skill, and professionalism are evident on every page of this book.

Julie Eckhert, my agent, friend, sounding board, cheerleader, and taskmaster. Thank you for all the recipes you contributed. More important, thank you for your guidance and support. None of this would have happened without you.

Lynne Drabkin, my mother-in-law, the best cook I have ever known, whose contributions to this book are too numerous to list. You went way beyond the call of duty!

Laura Marks, my wife and coauthor, who slaved in the kitchen for months while at the same time being the perfect mother, daughter, friend, pediatrician, and partner. Don't worry, we'll order in tonight!

—David R. Marks, M.D.

Note to All Headache Sufferers

THE IDEAS AND SUGGESTIONS in this book are not intended to substitute for a doctor's care. Anyone who suffers from headaches should be evaluated by a physician. This is especially important if you have the worst headache of your life, if your headache pain is different from your usual headache pattern, if the pain comes on rapidly and severely, if your headaches are accompanied by paralysis or slurred speech, or if you first develop headaches after fifty years of age.

Although this book describes effective steps to prevent headaches in many headache sufferers, it should not be used as a manual for self-diagnosis or self-treatment. All matters regarding your health require the consultation and supervision of a medical professional.

Contents

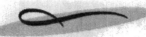

Foreword

I HAVE EXPERIENCED HEADACHES since I was a child. My mom has them. My grandmother had them. My aunts and uncles have them. My brother has them. We are basically a "headachy" family. But my headaches had always been infrequent and manageable—usually no more than three or four a month.

However, my headaches began to worsen and occur more frequently, perhaps due to increased stress. My family and friends worried that there was something seriously wrong. For months they encouraged me to see a doctor and get treatment; after all, I am the medical director of a world-renowned headache center! But, like many doctors who think they don't need help—and like many patients who mistakenly believe there is no remedy for their problem—I stubbornly refused to take my headaches seriously.

Finally, when I found myself taking more and more medication, I decided to treat myself the same way I treat my patients. For years I have counseled patients that certain foods can trigger headaches and urged them to avoid those foods, at least until the patients could determine whether those foods were the culprits. I put my patients on a headache-prevention diet, only to have them tell me that it was nearly impossible for them to find meals they liked while following the diet.

Luckily for me, however, my wife, Laura, is not only a doctor but also an excellent cook who loves to experiment in the kitchen. Together, we decided to create recipes that didn't rely on the headache-causing foods. And, naturally, we wanted these recipes to be delicious.

To satisfy our tastes, we included lots of easily prepared Italian and Mexican food, many delicious soups, and simple meat, poultry, and seafood dishes. I also have a major sweet tooth, so we came up with lots of mouthwatering, headache-friendly desserts.

After two weeks on the headache-prevention diet, my headaches began to improve. The longer I stayed on the diet, the better I felt, and within a month my life had completely changed for the better. The headaches that had become a major imposition were now only an occasional problem.

Although I have put patients on the headache-prevention diet in the past, I now do so with the conviction of someone whose life has been changed by it. Without the recipes that Laura developed, I would have scrapped the diet altogether, as many of my patients used to do.

Certainly, not all headaches are caused by food. Before embarking on the program in this book, you should be evaluated by a doctor to make sure that your headaches are not the symptom of a more serious condition. But I have seen countless patients who have been helped as much as I have by the headache-prevention diet. And until you eliminate the foods that have the potential to cause headaches and then gradually add them back, it is virtually impossible to determine whether your headaches are triggered, at least in part, by some of the foods you eat. This book can help you tackle your problem and lead you to a happier, pain-free life, while providing you with recipes for varied meals that aren't a headache to prepare.

Introduction

———

I F YOU'RE READING THIS, chances are that you or someone you know suffers from headaches. Take comfort in knowing that you're not alone! Headaches affect as many as 50 million Americans a year and account for more than 18 million visits to the doctor. In fact, headaches are the leading cause of absence from work; some researchers have estimated that 30 million workdays are lost each year because of the problem.

But numbers do not even begin to tell the story. The pain of a headache can completely disrupt a person's life. I have seen patients whose headaches are so severe that they are afraid to plan activities such as vacations, weddings, dinners, or dates. Their lives center on the dread of the next headache attack. Mary P. is a perfect example. When Mary came to my office, she had suffered from two to three headaches a week since her early twenties. Now that she was forty, her headaches were occurring on a daily basis. She complained of a constant throbbing sensation from the back of her head to her forehead. The headaches had become so severe that she was having difficulty taking care of her seven-year-old daughter and four-year-old son. The constant pain was also taking a toll on her marriage. The only way she could get through a day was by taking a lot of pain medicine.

Like Mary, many patients complain that their suffering is worsened by a feeling of helplessness. They have been told by friends and physicians alike that they will have to "learn to live with it." At one time or another, most headache sufferers have also been told, "It's all in your head." Often they blame themselves for their condition. The combination of fear, helplessness, and self-criticism can lead to depression and/or the chronic use of pain medication.

Many doctors now think that heredity may play a major part in the underlying cause of headaches. As I often tell my patients, if you really want to cure your headaches, you need to pick your parents better! I suspect that what a person inherits is the *predisposition* to getting headaches. I think of it like this: Everyone is born with a certain threshold for getting headaches. Some people have such a high threshold that they never get a headache, no matter how many "headache triggers" they are exposed to. Others have a headache threshold that is high enough so that they suffer from headaches only occasionally, and usually only with extreme triggers, such as severe stress or sleep deprivation. Frequent headache sufferers, on the other hand, are very sensitive to trigger factors and may get headaches in response to a multitude of them.

Headache Triggers

Stress, lack of sleep, bright lights, weather changes, and strong odors are all potential headache triggers. But what many people, including many doctors, don't realize is that some of the most common causes of headaches are ordinary foods that most of us eat every day. Avoiding those so-called food triggers can be one of the most effective and least invasive ways to treat headaches, without the risk of side effects and allergies (not to mention the cost) associated with the use of medications. In fact, by just following an appropriate headache-prevention diet, you may be able to get rid of most or all of your headaches!

You may still need to take medication for your pain. But medications have side effects—especially when they are taken too frequently. Indeed, one of the most frustrating things about treating headache patients is that they tend to be more sensitive to medications and experience more side effects than people without headaches. Whenever possible, it is ideal to be able to treat headaches without resorting to the use of medication. This is where diet modification is useful.

Diet modification worked for Mary P. After stopping her chronic pain medicines, we were able to identify many food triggers that she had previously been unaware of: Chinese food (even without MSG), cured pork products, aged cheeses, bananas, citrus fruits, and peanut butter cookies. Each of these foods caused a severe headache within hours of consumption. Once Mary identified her headache triggers, she modified her diet to avoid them. Her headaches became less frequent, and her relationships with her husband and children improved dramatically. Mary is just one person who has been helped by eliminating trigger foods from her diet. There are many others:

🌀 Indira P., a thirty-year-old Indian woman, moved to America in 1996 to make an arranged marriage. Shortly after her arrival, Indira developed headaches that occurred almost every day. But she spent the following winter in India and had no headaches while there. When she returned to the United States, her headaches recurred.

Indira did not believe that any of her headaches were caused by foods. However, I became suspicious after hearing that she had experienced no headaches while vacationing in India. I asked her what her husband did for a living. As it turns out, he operated a food truck that served sandwiches, and every day he would bring some home. Indira usually ate either a turkey and Swiss cheese or a cheese steak sandwich for lunch. I advised Indira to eliminate cheese from her diet, and when I saw her two months later her headaches were much better.

🌀 Sharon M. had daily headaches for about a year. The symptoms were typical of chronic tension-type headaches: a "tight band" around her head that was fairly constant and usually not associated with nausea or vomiting. After ruling out any serious cause of Sharon's headaches, I put her on the headache-prevention diet. Sharon kept a detailed record of everything she ate. (She is a bit compulsive, and in this case, it worked to her advantage.) When I next saw her two months later, she had experienced only a few headaches. Then, after slowly reintroducing the foods known to be common headache trig-

First, See a Doctor

Many people who see a doctor for their headaches do so because they are afraid that a brain tumor, an aneurysm, or another life-threatening problem is causing their pain. Fortunately, headaches that are related to some other medical problem, such as high blood pressure or an aneurysm, are relatively uncommon in people who are otherwise healthy and show no obvious signs of another medical problem. However, all headache sufferers should be thoroughly evaluated by a physician before it is assumed that their headaches are *not* due to a more serious condition. In some cases, a CT scan or an MRI (sophisticated X rays that let doctors see inside the brain) may be necessary to rule out a problem definitively.

Certain complaints make us worry that a headache may be caused by some underlying problem. Paying attention to these "red flags" is critical. Further evaluation may be warranted if a patient complains of having the worst headache of his or her life; if the headache pain is different from his or her usual headache pattern; if the pain comes on rapidly and severely (a "thunderclap headache"); if the person has neurological symptoms, such as paralysis, slurred speech, or loss of consciousness; or if the patient first develops headaches after fifty years of age.

gers, Sharon identified freshly baked bagels, pickles, chocolate, and citrus as some of her headache triggers. As a result, her life was, in her words, "totally changed."

John R. loved diet cola. At his initial evaluation, he said that he drank four glasses a day. Since diet cola contains artificial sweeten-

In most cases, even when a person has a red-flag symptom, we will still find nothing serious causing his or her headaches. But the consequences of missing something serious can be life-threatening and devastating.

One such patient was Mona C. She was sixty-four years old when she first came to my office. She began having headaches when she was eighteen, usually associated with her menstrual cycle. During menopause, her headaches decreased in frequency to three or four a year. But eight months prior to seeing me, Mona's headaches increased in frequency to at least a couple each month. This is not that unusual and would not necessarily have made me suspicious. However, the symptoms of her recent headaches differed from her usual pattern. Mona now had some mild visual distortion and dizziness associated with her headache pain. Neither of these was alarming in and of itself, but given her age, the sudden change in symptoms, and her feeling that the headaches just "weren't the same," I decided to order an MRI of her head.

The MRI revealed a large aneurysm in the right internal carotid artery—one of the main neck arteries leading to the brain. The aneurysm was located very close to the main artery that led to the right eye.

Mona needed urgent surgery. That test probably saved Mona's life.

ers and caffeine—both potential headache triggers—I recommended that he gradually reduce his intake and switch to something else. But, like many patients, John was reluctant to give up his favorite soft drink. He stopped drinking it for a short period of time, then tried to reintroduce it. Within hours, he suffered a severe migraine headache.

John tried on four more occasions to reintroduce diet cola. Each time ended with the same result: a migraine. Finally, he was forced to admit to himself that his favorite soft drink wasn't worth the pain.

🌀 Trisha P., age fifty-nine, suffered from headaches since she was eight. When Trisha first came to see me, she complained of frequent headaches and was taking too much pain medicine, which can cause "rebound" headaches. I discontinued her medication, and within a few short weeks, Trisha's headaches became much less frequent. To see if we could eliminate the rest of her headaches, I suggested that she avoid certain foods. After doing so for a few weeks, Trisha gradually began adding them back to her diet, one at a time, to try to identify the offenders. She reintroduced cheeses, artificial sweeteners, and pickles without any problems. One night, Trisha decided to have a piece of ice-cream cake with chocolate sprinkles on it. Seven hours later, she awakened with a migraine. Three days later, she ate a chocolate candy bar and developed a migraine within four hours. Since cutting chocolate out of her diet, Trisha has been doing fine, with only an occasional headache.

🌀 When I first saw Nancy R., she drank the equivalent of five cups of coffee a day. On top of that, she was taking a caffeine-containing pain medicine for her headaches on an almost daily basis. I warned her about the problems of "caffeine-rebound" headaches, but she insisted that she couldn't make it through a day without caffeine. After one year, Nancy's headaches became so severe that she began to feel desperate. Again I brought up the issue of her caffeine use, and we developed a plan: Nancy would stop her caffeine-containing pain medicine immediately and would begin tapering off her coffee intake, reducing it by one cup every three days until she had given up coffee completely. During the first couple of weeks off caffeine, Nancy had a number of bad headaches, but when I saw her a month later, her headaches had virtually disappeared.

Chocolate, caffeine, and red wine are common headache triggers, but as the stories of Mary, Indira, and John suggest, there are other, less well known offenders: most cheeses, citrus fruits, beans, freshly baked bread, artificial sweeteners, and preservatives, to name just a few. (A list of foods that frequently trigger headaches can be found on page 27.)

Not all these foods cause headaches all the time—most people are affected by only a small number of them. Some of my patients are unaffected by chocolate but will get a pounding headache from bananas.

🌀 Amy C. came to my office complaining of daily headaches that would get so bad that she had to close her office door and turn out the lights for hours at a time. Amy worked as a newswriter and producer, a high-stress position that regularly required twelve- to sixteen-hour workdays. She was not sleeping well, not exercising, and not eating properly. Amy skipped meals frequently, and when she did manage to eat, she ate as quickly as possible. She had gotten into the habit of eating bananas every day because of their convenience. Unfortunately for Amy, bananas are on the headache hit list, at least in large quantities. When Amy cut them out of her diet, her headaches improved.

🌀 Rhonda B.'s headaches, which used to trouble her only a few times a month, had become a daily torment. She had lost over forty pounds on a diet that prescribed eating three oranges and one grapefruit each day in addition to other low-fat foods. In Rhonda's case, it was the quantity of the citrus fruits that was the problem. Cutting back on her consumption of oranges and grapefruit helped keep her headaches in check.

🌀 Some people are affected by a particular food only at certain times. Eilene M., for example, was troubled by migraines around the time of menstruation. The migraines lasted for up to three days at a time, causing her to miss work. Eventually, Eilene noticed a pattern: Beginning about two days prior to her period and continuing until its end, eating bananas, grapefruit, or yogurt would cause her to develop a severe migraine within ten minutes. During the rest of the month, these foods did not affect her. Fortunately for Eilene, her menstrual cycle is regular, so she can avoid those food triggers during that time of the month.

Identifying Troublesome Foods

Not every headache sufferer is sensitive to food triggers. *The first step before undertaking any regimen is to see a doctor and determine if there is any underlying condition that may be causing your headaches.*

But a significant percentage of sufferers *are* affected by food, and I see it every day in my practice. Unfortunately, there is no physical sign or blood test that will tell you if some of your headaches are caused by food. And if you're not paying very close attention, you may not notice a pattern even if it's there. For that reason, I recommend that every headache sufferer try diet modification, at least temporarily. To discover if your diet is contributing to your headaches, you'll need to start with what doctors call an "elimination diet," in which you will try to eliminate all potentially troublesome foods (see page 27).

You can follow an elimination diet by using the recipes in this book and by creating your own recipes that avoid foods which can trigger headaches. You should avoid these foods for at least two months and record whether your headaches improve during this time.

After the two-month period, you can begin to reintroduce the potential trigger foods into your diet, one food at a time. Wait for a week or two before adding another. That way you can more accurately determine the effect of a particular food on your headache pattern. If your headaches increase after introducing a food, then you should assume it is a trigger and avoid it permanently. If the food does not result in any change in your headache pattern, you are not sensitive to it.

🌀 Paula S., a twenty-eight-year-old Italian woman, came to my office complaining of headaches that occurred three days a week. She was understandably distressed by their frequency but had noticed no particular pattern to them. Three weeks after starting the elimination diet, Paula's headaches improved dramatically. She was feeling great, but she wanted to go back to her normal diet. As Paula slowly began to reintroduce one food at a time, she remained headache-free, until she came to her favorite cheese-filled Italian foods: ziti with mozzarella, pizza, and lasagna, which she had previously indulged in several times a week—the same frequency with which she used to get headaches!

🌀 Another patient, Carla L., had discovered that she was sensitive to aged cheeses like cheddar and Parmesan. But when she ordered a chicken Caesar salad in a restaurant one day, it never occurred to her that the small amount of cheese in the dressing would be a problem. Big mistake! Within an hour, she developed a severe migraine.

Sometimes people have reactions to foods that don't usually cause headaches. These items are not included on the list of "forbidden" foods because they rarely cause problems. Unfortunately for some people, "rarely" is not the same as "never."

🌀 Gail H. was a teacher who went on the headache-prevention diet. One night she ate a lobster dinner. Within an hour, she developed a severe migraine. After that episode, Gail decided to experiment, and three days later, she had lobster bisque for lunch. Within an hour, she had a migraine. Because lobster is not a common headache trigger, it is not on the list of prohibited foods. But by paying careful attention to her headache pattern, Gail was able to determine that this food had an adverse effect on her.

🌀 Michael N.'s food reaction was one of the strangest I have seen in my practice. Michael never had a headache for the first thirty-five years of his life. One day, while driving, he bought a roll of hard butterscotch candies and put one in his mouth. Within fifteen minutes, Michael developed an excruciating cluster headache. He had trouble staying on the road but was able to make it to his destination. When he arrived, he was almost totally incapacitated. Fortunately, this attack lasted for only an hour and a half.

Headache Types

igraines, tension headaches, and cluster headaches, so classified because of their clinical symptoms, are the most common types of headaches. Unfortunately, there's no laboratory test to differentiate between these types of headaches. The correct diagnosis is important, however, because the treatment for each type can differ significantly. All three of these headaches can be triggered by foods.

Most headache specialists now believe that migraines and tension headaches are part of a continuum of headaches and share many similarities.

Migraine: The pain is typically described as a predominantly severe, throbbing, one-sided pain accompanied by nausea, vomiting, scalp tenderness, and extreme sensitivity to light and sound. Most people with migraines are debilitated during their headaches; indeed, migraines usually get worse with activity or exertion. For this reason, the migraine sufferer will usually prefer to lie down in a dark, quiet room until the headache ends, which can be anywhere from four hours to a few days. Nausea and vomiting can be so severe that intravenous (IV) fluids must be given in an emergency room.

About twenty percent of migraine sufferers experience an aura with their migraines. An aura is usually described as a visual condition in which a person sees brightly colored or wavy lines, flashing lights, or spots of different shapes and colors. The person may also have part of his or her visual field blacked out or may develop tunnel vision. Some people may have significant difficulty seeing at all. The aura develops quickly. It may occur before the migraine headache starts or may begin simultaneously with the headache.

Fortunately, aura symptoms generally disappear within an hour.

Tension Headache: In the past, this type of headache was called a "muscle-contraction" headache. It is the headache that most people are familiar with: Ninety percent of Americans will suffer this type of headache at least once in their lifetimes. Tension headaches are usually described as a squeezing or pressured sensation on the forehead, eyes, temples, or back of the head. Some people say their head "hurts all over." The pain is of mild to moderate intensity; it usually reduces but does not prohibit activity. Nausea without vomiting may be present; light or sound sensitivity is mild, if present at all. These headaches can last anywhere from thirty minutes to many days.

Cluster Headache: This Is an extremely painful condition; people have been known to commit suicide to escape their chronic suffering. The typical cluster headache is described as excruciating, sharp, stabbing, or burning and is usually felt in the eye or temple, as if someone is sticking a red-hot poker right through the eye to the back of the head. The headaches occur from one to ten times a day, last thirty minutes to two hours and are often accompanied by tearing and redness of the eye on the side of the headache, a drooping eye, and a runny or stuffy nose, also on the side of the headache.

The cluster headache has a unique pattern that seems to be tied to the body's biological clock. For example, cluster headaches often occur during sleep, and more than half of sufferers experience symptoms at about the same time each day. In most people, these headaches also seem to come and go in cycles during the year. A cycle may last from weeks to months, during which time the person will have frequent headaches. The rest of the year, the cluster sufferer is usually symptom-free. Then the cluster cycle may return at the same time the following year.

However, Michael did not make any association between his headaches and the butterscotch candy. Three days later he ate another butterscotch candy while driving his car. Once again, within fifteen minutes he had a severe cluster headache.

Why Do Certain Foods Trigger Headaches?

What is it about these foods that trigger headaches? There is certainly no factor common to all of these foods. The truth is that while theories abound, we are a long way from knowing what really causes the pain in your head. It is probably the result of a complex interaction between the nerves, blood vessels, and biochemicals located in the brain. The details of these interactions are unclear at present, but according to one theory, constriction of blood vessels to the brain decreases blood flow to the sensory area of the brain, resulting in the aura that often accompanies migraines. The blood vessels then expand, sending pulsations of blood to the brain, producing throbbing pain. Many headache specialists think that a neurochemical called serotonin plays a crucial role in bringing about these changes in blood vessels and other brain activity, altering blood flow and setting off a complicated cascade of events in the brain that results in a headache.

Food seems to be able to cause headaches regardless of whether you tend to get migraines, cluster headaches, or tension headaches. (For a discussion of the various kinds of headaches, see page 24.)

Although a few health-care practitioners maintain that allergies to certain foods set off headaches, most experts believe that such allergies play virtually no role in causing headaches. It is more likely that substances contained within some foods trigger the headaches either by changing the amount of serotonin in the brain or by affecting the blood vessels in the head. Amines, biochemicals involved in causing blood-vessel constriction and dilation, are found not only in the brain but in many different foods, such as cheese, chocolate, nuts, and certain meats. One common amine, called tyramine, is suspected by many experts to be a major factor in triggering headaches.

Preservatives such as nitrates and sulfites, artificial sweeteners such as aspartame and saccharin, and food additives such as monosodium glutamate (MSG) have all been implicated as headache triggers. They contain amines, which alter the constriction of the blood vessels. But for many of the foods listed below, the reason they trigger headaches remains a mystery. Scientists do know that alcohol can dilate blood vessels, and this may be one reason that alcohol can cause headaches. Many alcohols also contain amines such as tyramine and histamine. Caffeine can be a good treatment for headaches *when used in moderation.* Paradoxically, however, when it is taken on a daily basis, it can cause more headaches. Caffeine, in fact, is one of the most common food-related causes of headaches that I see in my practice, and it's the one thing patients often have the most resistance to giving up, until they discover that doing so can help them eliminate disabling pain.

Using This Book

All the recipes in this book have been created without using the major ingredients that are known to be headache triggers. We have noted which foods should be eaten in only small quantities and have tried to suggest the appropriate limits.

We encourage you to add your own headache recipes to ours. We would love to hear about them so we can share them with other patients. By doing so, you will be helping a fellow headache sufferer.

Headache-Causing Foods

The list of foods that have been reported to trigger headaches is long and varied. The foods included here are the ones most commonly reported to cause headaches; that's why it's difficult to avoid them without following the headache-prevention diet. Some of you may be susceptible to many of these foods, others to only a few. If you are lucky, you'll find you're not susceptible to any of these foods. The only way to tell is by going on the headache-prevention diet. If you discover an ingredient that triggers your headaches and is not on this list, you should obviously avoid it too.

VEGETABLES

Prohibited: Beans (lima, Italian, pole, broad, fava, string, navy, pinto, garbanzo, lentils, snow peas), pickles, chili peppers, olives.

Allowed: All other fresh, frozen, dried, and canned vegetables and vegetable juices. Limit tomatoes to ½ cup per day; limit onions to ½ cup per day.

FRUITS

Prohibited: Dried fruits that contain preservatives (such as raisins, dates, figs, apricots), avocados, papayas, passion fruit, red plums, banana-peel extract.

Allowed: All other fresh, frozen, and canned fruits and juices. Limit citrus fruits (oranges, grapefruits, tangerines, lemons, limes) and pineapple to ½ cup per day. Limit bananas to ½ banana per day. (Technically, a tomato is a fruit, so remember to limit tomatoes to ½ cup per day.) Organic dried fruits without preservatives (particularly sulfites).

BREADS AND CEREALS

Prohibited: Any fresh yeast product straight out of the oven; for example, yeast breads, crackers, pizza dough, doughnuts, soft pretzels.

Allowed: Store-bought and homemade breads (white, whole wheat, French, Italian, bagels, etc.) are fine as long as they are not straight out of the oven and have been allowed to cool (it's OK to reheat them). Just be careful that they don't contain other prohibited ingredients, such as raisins, nuts, chocolate, or cheeses. Likewise, you can eat all hot and cold cereals unless they contain specifically prohibited items, such as dried fruit or artificial sweeteners.

DAIRY PRODUCTS AND EGGS

Prohibited: Most cheeses. Sour cream, whole milk, chocolate milk, buttermilk, cream.

Allowed: Skim milk or 1% homogenized milk. Cheeses: American, ricotta, cream cheese, Velveeta, pot, farmer, cottage. Skim milk–based yogurt (limit it to ½ cup per day). Eggs.

BEVERAGES

Prohibited: Alcoholic beverages, especially red wine; beverages containing chocolate or cocoa; diet beverages containing artificial sweeteners.

Allowed: Fruit and vegetable juices, noncaffeinated drinks (if they don't contain artificial sweeteners). Limit caffeinated drinks, such as coffee, tea, or soda, to 2 cups (approximately 16 ounces) per day. For soda, that's a little more than one can a day.

SOUPS

Prohibited: Most canned soups and bouillon cubes (they usually contain MSG, preservatives, or other prohibited ingredients).

Allowed: Homemade soups and stocks, unless they contain other specifically prohibited foods, such as beans, cheese, or large amounts of onion or tomato.

DESSERTS

Prohibited: Chocolate, carob, and licorice; ice cream; desserts containing other prohibited foods, such as nuts or dried fruit, or those made with liqueurs; whipped cream.

Allowed: Cakes, cookies, candies, and pies, unless they contain prohibited ingredients; gelatin, sherbet, and sorbet.

MISCELLANEOUS

Prohibited: Monosodium glutamate (MSG) and tenderizers containing MSG; soy sauce; vinegar, except for white and cider vinegars; salad dressings containing wine or vinegar, unless it is white or cider vinegar; cooking sherry; olive oil; seeds, nuts, peanuts, and peanut butter; all artificial sweeteners; preservatives, such as nitrates and sulfites; coconuts; capers. Most mustards, ketchups, and mayonnaises.

Allowed: Anything else not specifically prohibited, all herbs and spices, white vinegar, cider vinegar, honey, jams, jellies, dry mustard.

MEAT AND SEAFOOD

Prohibited: Bacon, hot dogs, pepperoni, sausage, salami, bologna, ham; organs (liver and other organ meats); all aged, canned, cured, or processed meat products; caviar.

Allowed: All fresh beef, poultry, fish, or pork products, unless specifically prohibited; tuna and other canned seafood that is packed in water.

Breakfast and Brunch

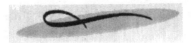

Orange Blossom French Toast

SERVES 2

An unexpected burst of orange flavors this morning standard,
which is also served with an orange sauce.
Our kids look forward to having this on Sunday mornings.

3 **large eggs**
   Rind of 1 orange, finely grated
⅓ **cup orange juice**
½ **teaspoon orange extract**
6 **slices day-old white bread**
2 **large navel oranges**
2 **tablespoons (¼ stick) unsalted butter**
1 **tablespoon light brown sugar**
2 **tablespoons canola oil**

Beat together the eggs, orange zest, juice, and orange extract in a baking dish large enough to hold the bread slices in a single layer. Dip both sides of each bread slice into the egg mixture. Arrange the bread slices in a single layer in the dish and let the bread soak up all the egg mixture, about 10 minutes.

Meanwhile, peel the oranges, being careful to remove all the white membrane around the outside. Using a sharp knife, separate the oranges into sections, cutting between the inner membranes. Discard the membranes and any accumulated juice.

Melt 1 tablespoon of the butter and the brown sugar in a small saucepan over low heat. When the mixture foams, add the orange sections and cook, stirring, just until heated through, about 3 minutes. Remove the orange sauce from the heat, cover, and keep warm.

Heat the oil in a large skillet or brush it onto a large griddle over medium heat. Add the remaining 1 tablespoon butter. When the butter foams, add the bread slices and cook until golden brown, turning once, about 5 minutes per side. Serve immediately with the orange sauce.

Crunchy French Toast

SERVES 2

This variation on the classic breakfast dish
turns French toast into a spectacular meal.

3 large eggs
⅓ cup skim milk
½ teaspoon vanilla extract
6 slices day-old white bread
1 cup corn flakes
2 tablespoons canola oil
1 tablespoon unsalted butter
   Pure maple syrup, warmed

Beat together the eggs, milk, and vanilla extract in a baking dish large enough to hold the bread slices in a single layer. Dip both sides of each bread slice into the egg mixture. Arrange the bread slices in a single layer in the dish and let the bread soak up all the egg mixture, about 10 minutes.

Transfer the bread slices to a large plate. Cover the bottom of the baking dish with the corn flakes. Return the bread slices to the baking dish and press them gently into the corn flakes. Turn the bread slices, trying not to dislodge the corn flakes, and press the corn flakes into the other side.

Heat the oil in a large skillet or brush it onto a large griddle over medium heat. Add the butter. When the butter foams, add the bread slices and cook until golden brown, turning once, about 5 minutes per side. Serve immediately with the syrup.

Hearty Potato-Mushroom Frittata

SERVES 6

Many frittatas contain ingredients that are forbidden on the headache-prevention diet—especially cured meats, such as bacon, ham, and sausage. This flavorful frittata is made without any trigger foods. It's substantial enough for a light supper.

- 2 **tablespoons (¼ stick) butter**
- 12 **ounces white button mushrooms, sliced**
  Salt and freshly ground pepper
- 2 **tablespoons canola oil**
- 4 **medium russet potatoes, baked, cooled, peeled, and sliced**
- ¾ **cup coarsely chopped fresh basil**
- 12 **large eggs**

Preheat the oven to 400 degrees F.

Heat the butter in a large skillet over medium heat. Add the mushrooms, and sauté, stirring occasionally, for 10 minutes, or until softened. Season with salt and pepper to taste. Brush a 13-x-9-inch baking dish with the oil. Layer half of the potato slices in the bottom of the dish. Season with salt and pepper to taste. Layer half of the basil and then half of the mushrooms into the dish. Repeat with the remaining potato slices, then the remaining basil, and the remaining mushrooms.

Beat the eggs in a large bowl and season with salt and pepper to taste. Pour the eggs evenly over the vegetables in the baking dish. Bake for 20 minutes, or until the eggs are set and puffy and the top is golden brown. (A toothpick inserted into the center of the frittata should come out clean.) Serve hot or at room temperature.

Lacy Potato Pancakes with Applesauce

MAKES ABOUT 3 DOZEN PANCAKES; SERVES 6 TO 8

Our whole family looks forward to Hanukkah every year—not for the presents but for these potato pancakes, or latkes, as they're called in Yiddish. They also make great hors d'oeuvres.

APPLESAUCE

4–5   **Granny Smith apples, peeled, cored, and cut into large pieces**
⅓   **cup boiling water**
½   **cup sugar**

POTATO PANCAKES

2½   **pounds russet potatoes, peeled**
1   **small onion**
1   **large egg, lightly beaten**
1   **tablespoon all-purpose flour**
   Salt and freshly ground pepper
   Canola oil

APPLESAUCE: Place the apples and water in a medium saucepan and boil for 12 to 15 minutes, or until the apples can be mashed easily with a fork. Stir in the sugar and cook until it dissolves, about 5 minutes. Pour the apple mixture into a food processor and pulse until smooth. Transfer to a medium bowl, set aside, and keep warm. Rinse the food processor and blade.

POTATO PANCAKES: Puree half of the potatoes and the onion in the food processor. Transfer the potato mixture to a large bowl.

Shred the remaining potatoes in the food processor, using the shredding blade. Add to the potato-onion mixture, then drain off and reserve the liquid from the potato-mixture bowl. Add the egg, flour, and salt and pepper to taste to the potato mixture; it should have the consistency of sour cream. If it is too thin, add a bit more flour; if it is too thick, add some of the reserved potato liquid.

Heat 1 inch of oil in a large skillet over medium-high heat to 400 degrees F. A cube of bread tossed in should sizzle and brown. Line a large platter with paper towels. Drop heaping tablespoons of the potato mixture into the skillet; do not crowd. Flatten the pancakes with the back of the spoon and fry in batches, turning once, until golden brown, about 5 minutes per side. Transfer the pancakes to the paper-towel-lined platter to drain. Continue until all the potato mixture is used, adding more oil if necessary.

Serve the potato pancakes with the warm applesauce on the side.

Spinach Pie

SERVES 8 TO 10

The original recipe for this spinach pie contained cheddar and mozzarella, but in deference to David's headaches, Laura's mother substituted cream cheese and added garlic and tarragon to boost the flavor.

4 large eggs
6 ounces cream cheese, at room temperature
¼ cup plus 2 tablespoons all-purpose flour
¼ cup skim milk
2 tablespoons (¼ stick) butter, at room temperature
1 teaspoon minced garlic
1 teaspoon dried tarragon, crumbled
1 teaspoon salt
⅛ teaspoon cayenne pepper
⅛ teaspoon freshly ground black pepper
1 16-ounce bag frozen chopped spinach, thawed, water squeezed out
1 frozen unbaked pie shell

Preheat the oven to 325 degrees F.

Beat together the eggs, cream cheese, flour, milk, butter, garlic, tarragon, salt, cayenne, and pepper in a large bowl. Fold in the spinach.

Pour the mixture into the pie shell and bake for 25 minutes, or until the filling is set and the crust is golden brown. Serve hot or at room temperature.

Spinach and Cheese Strata

SERVES 6 TO 8

Velveeta cheese ensures that this dish is safe for the headache sufferer.
Our kids love it.

12 ¾-inch slices Italian or French bread
    (without seeds)
 8 ounces Velveeta cheese, shredded
 1 16-ounce package frozen chopped spinach, thawed,
    water squeezed out
 1 tablespoon butter
1½ cups skim milk
 3 large eggs
 ½ cup chopped fresh basil
 ½ teaspoon salt
 ¼ teaspoon freshly ground pepper

Spray a 13-x-9-inch baking dish with cooking spray. Arrange half of the bread slices in a single layer in the dish. Top the bread with half of the cheese. Layer the spinach over the cheese, then top with the remaining cheese.

Butter one side of each remaining bread slice and place the slices, buttered side up, in a single layer on top of the cheese.

Whisk together the milk, eggs, basil, salt, and pepper in a medium bowl. Pour the egg mixture evenly over the top of the bread slices. Prick the bread slices with a fork in many places to help them absorb the egg mixture. Cover the baking dish with plastic wrap and let stand in the refrigerator for at least 30 minutes or overnight.

Preheat the oven to 350 degrees F.

Remove the plastic wrap and bake for 1 hour, or until a knife inserted into the center of the strata comes out clean. Serve immediately.

Crepes with Spinach and Cheese Filling

SERVES 8

These light, tender crepes with a melt-in-your-mouth spinach filling are perfect for brunch. Crepes are one of the most versatile items in a cook's repertoire. They can be used to enhance leftovers or to create a party dish out of everyday ingredients.

SPINACH AND CHEESE FILLING

1   16-ounce bag frozen chopped spinach, thawed, water squeezed out
8   ounces cream cheese, at room temperature
8   ounces part-skim ricotta cheese
2   large eggs
2   teaspoons salt
½   teaspoon freshly ground pepper

CREPES

8   tablespoons (1 stick) unsalted butter
3   large eggs
1   cup all-purpose flour
⅔   cup skim milk
⅔   cup cold water
¼   teaspoon salt

About 3 tablespoons melted butter

FILLING : Whisk the spinach, cream cheese, ricotta cheese, eggs, salt, and pepper in a large bowl until thoroughly combined. Set aside in the refrigerator.

CREPES : Melt the butter in a small saucepan over low heat. Spoon off and discard the foam from the top. Pour off the clarified butter into a small bowl and discard the solids in the bottom of the pan. You should have about 6 tablespoons clarified butter.

Whisk together the clarified butter, eggs, flour, milk, water, and salt in a medium bowl. Let the batter stand for 1 hour in the refrigerator.

Spray a crepe pan lightly with cooking spray. Set the pan over medium heat just until it begins to smoke. Pour about ¼ cup of the batter into the pan. Quickly swirl the pan to cover the bottom with batter. Pour any batter that does not stick to the pan back into the bowl.

Cook the crepe for approximately 1 minute, or until the bottom is light brown. Flip the crepe over and brown the other side briefly. (The first crepe may not be perfect, but the rest should be fine.) Repeat with the remaining batter.

Stack the crepes on a plate, placing a piece of wax paper between each crepe.

Preheat the oven to 350 degrees F.

ASSEMBLY : Fill each crepe with ¼ cup of the spinach mixture. Roll up the crepes and place them seam side down in a 13-x-9-inch baking dish sprayed lightly with cooking spray. Cover the dish with aluminum foil and bake until the filling is heated through, about 20 minutes. Drizzle about ½ teaspoon of the melted butter over each crepe and serve hot.

Crepes with Chicken and Mushroom Filling

SERVES 4 AS A MAIN DISH, 8 AS AN APPETIZER

These crepes can be served as a main course or
as an appetizer. The béchamel sauce that coats the crepes
keeps them moist and flavorful.

CHICKEN AND MUSHROOM FILLING

1   pound boneless, skinless chicken breasts
4   tablespoons (½ stick) butter
1   tablespoon canola oil
¼   cup finely diced shallots
6   ounces white button mushrooms, minced
1¼ cups homemade chicken stock (page 58)
2½ tablespoons all-purpose flour
½   cup skim milk, heated
    Salt and freshly ground pepper
    Fresh lemon juice

Crepes (page 40)

½   cup fresh bread crumbs

FILLING: Place the chicken breasts in a medium saucepan with just enough water to cover. Bring to a simmer over high heat, then reduce the heat to low, cover, and cook until the juices run clear when the chicken is pierced with a fork, 20 to 25 minutes. Remove from the water with a slotted spoon and let cool slightly. Dice the chicken and set aside.

Heat 2 tablespoons of the butter and the oil in a large skillet over medium heat. Add the shallots and sauté, stirring occasionally, until translucent, about 5 minutes. Add the mushrooms and sauté, stirring, until tender, about 5 minutes. Stir in the diced chicken, reduce the heat to low, and cook until the chicken is heated through. Transfer to a medium bowl and keep warm.

Add ¼ cup of the stock to the skillet, increase the heat to medium, and bring to a boil, scraping up the brown bits from the bottom of the skillet. Add the remaining 2 tablespoons butter. When the butter melts, stir in the flour and cook, stirring, until the flour mixture is light brown, about 2 minutes. Slowly add the remaining 1 cup stock and the milk, stirring constantly. Cook, stirring frequently, until the sauce is thick enough to coat a spoon, 8 to 10 minutes more. Season with salt, pepper, and lemon juice to taste. Remove sauce from the heat.

C R E P E S : Make the crepes as directed on page 41.

A S S E M B L Y : Preheat the broiler. Stir ¾ cup of the sauce into the chicken mixture. Fill each crepe with a heaping tablespoon of the chicken mixture. Roll up the crepes and place them seam side down in a broilerproof 13-x-9-inch baking dish sprayed lightly with cooking spray. Spread the remaining sauce over the crepes and sprinkle with the bread crumbs. Broil until the crepes are browned, about 3 minutes, watching carefully so they don't burn. Serve hot.

Appetizers

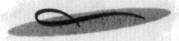

Garlic Artichoke Toasts

MAKES 16 TRIANGLES; SERVES 8

David and I love artichokes, but our favorite artichoke dip
contained two kinds of cheese that can trigger headaches.
I was determined to create a headache-safe version.
This is even better than our old favorite.

3   **whole garlic heads (not cloves)**
1   **tablespoon canola oil**
2   **ounces cream cheese, at room temperature**
1   **14-ounce can water-packed artichoke hearts**
2   **teaspoons melted butter**
1   **teaspoon fresh lemon juice**
½   **teaspoon dried cilantro, crumbled**
½   **teaspoon salt**
¼   **teaspoon freshly ground pepper**
8   **thin slices white sandwich bread, toasted,
    crusts removed**

Preheat the oven to 350 degrees F.

Cut off and discard the top ⅛ inch from the garlic heads. Place each
garlic head on a square of aluminum foil large enough to enclose it and
drizzle the oil over the garlic. Wrap the foil over the garlic and place on
a cookie sheet. Bake for 30 minutes, or until the garlic is softened.

Let the garlic cool slightly, then squeeze the garlic cloves out of the
skins into a food processor. Pulse until the garlic is coarsely chopped.
Add the cream cheese and process until thoroughly combined. Transfer
the garlic mixture to a small bowl and set aside.

Place the artichoke hearts in the food processor and pulse until coarsely chopped. Transfer to a separate small bowl and stir in the butter, lemon juice, cilantro, salt, and pepper.

Spread the garlic mixture on the pieces of toast and top with the artichoke mixture. Cut each piece of toast in half diagonally. Place the toasts on a large plate and heat in a microwave on high power for 30 seconds, or until heated through. Alternatively, preheat the oven to 350 degrees F. Place the toasts on a cookie sheet and bake for 5 minutes, or until heated through. Serve hot or warm.

Eggplant "Caviar"

SERVES 6 TO 8

The small amounts of tomato and onion in each serving should cause no problems unless you eat too much—a distinct possibility once you've tasted this hors d'oeuvre.

- 1 **medium eggplant**
- 1 **medium tomato, seeded and chopped**
- ½ **cup minced onion**
- 3 **tablespoons canola oil**
- 2 **tablespoons fresh lemon juice**
- 1 **garlic clove, minced**
- 1 **teaspoon sugar**
   Salt and freshly ground pepper

Crackers or buttered rounds of toasted rye bread

Preheat the oven to 400 degrees F.

Place the eggplant in a small baking dish and bake for 30 minutes, or until soft. Let the eggplant cool, then peel it and finely chop the flesh in a food processor or by hand. Place the eggplant in a medium bowl and stir in the tomato, onion, oil, lemon juice, garlic, sugar, and salt and pepper to taste. Refrigerate until cold. Spread the eggplant mixture on the crackers or toasts and serve.

Ricotta Puffs

MAKES ABOUT 3 DOZEN PUFFS; SERVES 12

Ricotta cheese makes these deep-fried puffs light and airy.
There's just a little sun-dried tomato in each puff—well
below the recommended limit.

3 cups canola oil
1 15-ounce container nonfat ricotta cheese
1 cup all-purpose flour
2 large eggs
1 teaspoon baking powder
1 10-ounce package frozen chopped spinach, thawed,
    water squeezed out
¾ cup chopped dry-packed sun-dried tomatoes,
    soaked in hot water for 10 minutes and drained
2 teaspoons salt
½ teaspoon dried oregano, crumbled
¼ teaspoon crushed red pepper flakes

Heat the oil in a deep skillet over medium-high heat to 375 degrees
F. A cube of bread tossed into the oil will sizzle and brown. Line a large
plate with paper towels.

Combine the ricotta cheese, flour, eggs, and baking powder in a
large bowl. Add the spinach, sun-dried tomatoes, salt, oregano, and red
pepper flakes and mix until the ingredients are evenly distributed.

With your hands, roll 1 level teaspoon of the ricotta mixture into
a ball. Repeat with the remaining ricotta mixture. With a slotted
spoon, carefully add the ricotta balls to the hot oil. The puffs will turn
golden brown quickly, about 5 minutes. Turn and let the other side
brown slightly. Drain on the paper-towel-lined plate. Serve hot.

Sautéed Mushrooms on Toast

SERVES 4

This creation satisfies my love of mushrooms.
It's a big hit with our friends.

3 tablespoons butter
1 tablespoon canola oil
16 ounces white button mushrooms,
    stems trimmed, sliced
¼ cup chopped fresh parsley
1 tablespoon fresh lemon juice
1 garlic clove, minced
½ teaspoon salt
⅛ teaspoon freshly ground pepper
4 slices white sandwich bread, crusts removed

Heat 2 tablespoons of the butter and the oil in a large skillet over medium heat. Add the mushrooms, parsley, lemon juice, garlic, salt, and pepper. Cook, stirring occasionally, for 5 minutes, or until the mushrooms release their juice.

Meanwhile, spread some of the remaining 1 tablespoon butter on both sides of the bread slices. Heat a large skillet over medium-high heat and sauté the bread slices until golden brown, about 3 minutes per side. Cut each slice in half diagonally and place in a serving dish. Spoon the mushroom mixture over the pan-toasted bread and serve.

Spinach-Stuffed Mushrooms

MAKES 12 MUSHROOMS; SERVES 6

The creamy filling of these stuffed mushrooms
uses no forbidden cheeses. The recipe comes from
David's friend and agent, Julie Eckhert.

1   **10-ounce package frozen leaf spinach**
2   **tablespoons cream cheese, at room temperature**
    Pinch ground nutmeg
    Pinch salt
3   **teaspoons butter**
1   **scallion, chopped**
12 **large white button mushrooms**

Cook the spinach according to the package directions and drain thoroughly. Transfer the spinach to a medium bowl and stir in the cream cheese, nutmeg, and salt. Set aside.

Meanwhile, heat 1 teaspoon of the butter in a small skillet over medium heat. Add the scallion and sauté, stirring, until lightly browned, about 2 minutes. Transfer the scallion and the spinach mixture to a food processor and puree.

Remove and discard the stems from the mushrooms and scrape out any parts of the stems that remain in the caps. Stuff the mushroom caps with the spinach mixture.

Grease a cookie sheet with 1 teaspoon of the butter. Preheat the broiler. Place the stuffed mushrooms on the cookie sheet. Melt the remaining 1 teaspoon butter in a small skillet over low heat and brush it on the mushrooms. Broil until the mushrooms are lightly browned, about 5 minutes. Serve immediately.

Portobello Mushrooms Stuffed with Cream Cheese and Sun-Dried Tomatoes

SERVES 8

This appetizer is a favorite at parties. Be careful: If you overindulge, you'll risk exceeding the limit on tomatoes.

5 **tablespoons canola oil**
½ **cup finely chopped shallots**
3 **garlic cloves, minced**
¾ **cup chopped dry-packed sun-dried tomatoes,**
   soaked in hot water for 10 minutes and drained
2 **teaspoons dried basil, crumbled**
1 **teaspoon salt**
½ **teaspoon crushed red pepper flakes**
½ **cup chopped fresh flat-leaf parsley**
8 **ounces cream cheese, at room temperature**
8 **portobello mushrooms**

Heat 2 tablespoons of the oil in a large skillet over medium heat. Sauté the shallots, stirring occasionally, until browned, about 4 minutes. Add the garlic and sauté for 2 minutes more, then add the sun-dried tomatoes, basil, salt, and red pepper flakes and cook, stirring occasionally, for 4 minutes more, or until heated through. Remove from the heat and stir in the parsley.

Combine the cream cheese and 1 tablespoon of the oil in a small bowl. Add to the sun-dried-tomato mixture and mix well.

Remove and discard the stems from the mushrooms. Brush the mushrooms generously with the remaining 2 tablespoons oil.

Heat a large skillet over medium heat until a drop of cold water sputters on the surface. Add the mushrooms to the skillet stem side down and cook for 4 minutes, or until tender. Turn and cook for 2 minutes more, or until tender when pierced with a fork.

Arrange the mushrooms stem side up on a serving platter and fill each mushroom cap with a generous amount of the cheese mixture. Serve warm.

Asparagus Roll-Ups

MAKES 25 ROLL-UPS; SERVES 8

I like to serve this appetizer at parties . . .
if David doesn't finish them off before the guests arrive.

25 **medium asparagus spears, ends snapped off,
    halved crosswise**
8 **tablespoons (1 stick) unsalted butter**
4 **large egg yolks**
2 **tablespoons fresh lemon juice**
½ **teaspoon salt**
¼ **teaspoon dry mustard**
   Pinch cayenne pepper
25 **thin slices white sandwich bread**

Cook the asparagus in a large saucepan of boiling water until crisp-tender, about 3 minutes. Drain the asparagus and shock it in an ice-water bath. Drain again and set aside.

Melt the butter in a small saucepan over medium heat until hot. Combine the egg yolks, lemon juice, salt, mustard, and cayenne in a food processor and process until frothy. With the motor running, gradually add the butter in a thin stream to the food processor and process until blended. Set aside.

With a diamond-shaped cookie cutter, cut out diamonds from the centers of the bread slices; reserve the remaining bread for another use. With a rolling pin, roll out the diamonds of bread until thin.

Preheat the broiler.

Spread each diamond of bread with the lemon sauce, using a total of about two-thirds of the sauce. Place 2 asparagus halves (1 top and 1 bottom) on each bread diamond. Bring 2 opposite corners of each diamond together to wrap the asparagus and fasten the overlapping corners with a toothpick. Dot the tops of the roll-ups with more of the sauce. Place the roll-ups on a cookie sheet and broil until the tops of the bread are crisp; about 5 minutes. Serve warm.

Endive with Herbed Cream Cheese

MAKES APPROXIMATELY 2 DOZEN; SERVES 8

The original recipe contained blue cheese, but this headache-safe mix of cream cheese and herbs is every bit as good.

8 ounces cream cheese, at room temperature
1 tablespoon butter, at room temperature
2 garlic cloves
¼ teaspoon fresh lemon juice
¼ teaspoon dried tarragon, crumbled
¼ teaspoon dried thyme, crumbled
¼ teaspoon dried basil, crumbled
¼ teaspoon dried oregano, crumbled
¼ teaspoon salt
Pinch cayenne pepper
½ teaspoon water
2 heads endive, separated into leaves
1 cup alfalfa sprouts

Place the cream cheese and butter in a food processor and pulse to combine. Add the garlic, lemon juice, tarragon, thyme, basil, oregano, salt, and cayenne and process until thoroughly combined. Add the water, ¼ teaspoon at a time, while pulsing the food processor. Transfer the cream-cheese mixture to a medium bowl and let the mixture sit at room temperature for 1 hour. (You can make the cream-cheese mixture up to 3 days ahead, cover, and refrigerate.)

With a teaspooon, spread about ¾ teaspoon of the cream-cheese mixture onto the bottom half of each endive leaf. Sprinkle a few alfalfa sprouts over each leaf. Arrange the leaves on a platter and serve cold.

Soups

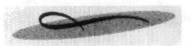

Mom's Chicken Stock

MAKES 6 CUPS

If chicken soup has healing properties, then this stock
is the best medicine of all for headache sufferers.
Use in place of canned broth or bouillon cubes, which often
contain MSG or other headache-producing additives.

1   4-to-5-pound chicken, quartered
2   quarts water
6   large carrots, peeled and cut into large pieces
2   medium onions, halved
1½ teaspoons salt
1½ teaspoons freshly ground pepper

Combine all the ingredients in a large pot. Bring to a boil, skimming off any foam. Reduce the heat to low, cover partially, and simmer for 1½ hours. Let the stock cool to room temperature. Strain the stock into a large bowl. Discard the vegetables, and skin and bone the chicken. Reserve the chicken meat for another use. Refrigerate the stock until the fat congeals. Skim off and discard the fat. The stock may be frozen in ice-cube trays for up to 3 months and used in recipes as needed.

Beef Stock

MAKES 6 CUPS

Use this homemade stock in place of canned beef broth, which often contains headache-triggering ingredients.

3 **pounds beef short ribs**
2 **quarts water**
1 **pound carrots, peeled and cut into 2-inch pieces**
1 **large onion, quartered**
1½ **teaspoons salt**
¼ **teaspoon freshly ground pepper**

Combine all the ingredients in a large pot. Bring to a boil, skimming off any foam. Reduce the heat to low, cover partially, and simmer, occasionally skimming off any foam, for 2½ to 3 hours, or until the meat is tender and the stock is flavorful. Let the stock cool to room temperature. Remove the beef, carrots, and onions and reserve for another use or discard.

Refrigerate the stock until the fat congeals. Skim off and discard the fat. The stock may be frozen in ice-cube trays for up to 3 months and used in recipes as needed.

Homemade Vegetable Stock

MAKES 8 TO 9 CUPS

You can change the character of this stock by
adding different vegetables to the mix.
Serve the stock on its own or use as a base for soups and sauces.

3   quarts water
6   large carrots, peeled and chopped
4   large celery stalks, chopped
1   bunch scallions, chopped
     Any fresh vegetables you wish to add, such as
        mushrooms, turnips, potatoes, corn, parsnips,
        or sweet potatoes
5   garlic cloves, minced
3   sprigs fresh parsley
2   bay leaves
¼   teaspoon dried thyme, crumbled
⅛   teaspoon ground cloves
     Salt to taste

Combine all the ingredients in a large pot. Bring to a boil, reduce
the heat to low, cover partially, and simmer for 3 to 4 hours, or until
the stock is flavorful. If the stock is too strong, add more water to taste.
Let the stock cool to room temperature. Strain into a large bowl; discard the vegetables. The stock may be frozen in ice-cube trays for up to
3 months and used in recipes as needed.

Corn and Carrot Chowder

SERVES 4

Served with bread, this delicious chowder
makes a great lunch or light dinner.

2	medium potatoes, peeled and cut into ½-inch cubes
	Salt
2½	tablespoons butter
½	cup chopped scallions
2½	cups 1% milk
1	10-ounce package frozen corn or 1¾ cups fresh corn kernels
2	large carrots, peeled and thinly sliced
1	4-ounce jar pimientos, drained and chopped
1	tablespoon light brown sugar
¼	teaspoon paprika
	Pinch dried thyme, crumbled
	Freshly ground pepper

Place the potatoes in a large pot and add just enough water to cover and salt to taste. Bring to a boil, reduce the heat to medium, and simmer for 15 minutes, or until barely tender. Pour off about half of the water and reduce the heat to low.

Meanwhile, melt the butter in a small skillet over medium-high heat. Add the scallions and sauté, stirring, until soft, about 5 minutes. Add the scallions, milk, corn, carrots, pimientos, brown sugar, paprika, thyme, and salt and pepper to taste to the potatoes. Simmer for about 30 minutes, stirring occasionally, until the chowder is thickened to the desired consistency. Serve hot.

Roasted Vegetable Soup

SERVES 8

The amount of tomatoes in this hearty soup is within the parameters of the headache-prevention diet. If you're sensitive to onions, leave them out. Carol Bronz, a nurse at Norwalk Hospital in Norwalk, Connecticut, contributed this recipe.

2   large eggplants, peeled and cut into
    1-inch-thick rounds
4   medium red bell peppers, stemmed, halved,
    and seeded
4   medium tomatoes, cored
3   large carrots, peeled and halved lengthwise
3   small zucchini, peeled and halved lengthwise
1   medium fennel bulb, trimmed and halved
4   tablespoons (½ stick) butter
3   medium onions, sliced
5–6   garlic cloves
3–4   cups homemade chicken stock (page 58)
    Salt and freshly ground pepper
    Pinch cayenne pepper
¼   cup chopped fresh basil

Preheat the oven to 400 degrees F.

Place the eggplant, red peppers, tomatoes, carrots, zucchini, and fennel on a cookie sheet lined with aluminum foil. Roast until the vegetables are softened, removing each vegetable as it is done, about 40 minutes for the tomatoes and red peppers, 50 minutes for the eggplant and zucchini, and 1 hour for the carrots and fennel. Remove and discard any charred skin from the tomatoes and red peppers.

Meanwhile, heat the butter in a large pot over medium heat. Add the onions and sauté, stirring, until golden brown, about 15 minutes. Add the garlic and sauté until garlic is softened, about 3 minutes more.

Add the roasted vegetables to the pot, along with enough stock to barely cover them. Season with salt and pepper to taste and add the cayenne. Bring to a boil over high heat, reduce the heat to low, cover partially, and simmer for 30 minutes, or until the vegetables are very soft. Puree the soup in a blender. Return the soup to the pot and thin to the desired consistency with more stock, if needed. Stir in the basil and serve hot.

Cream of Three-Mushroom Soup

SERVES 8

Dr. Alan Rapoport, David's colleague at the New England Center for Headache and a mushroom-soup connoisseur, pronounced this version the best he's ever tasted.

4   tablespoons (½ stick) butter
3   medium onions, sliced
8   garlic cloves, minced
24   ounces white button mushrooms, stemmed
10   ounces cremini mushrooms, stemmed
10   ounces portobello mushrooms, stemmed
    About 3 cups homemade chicken stock (page 58)
1   12-ounce can evaporated skim milk
    Salt and freshly ground pepper
1   tablespoon chopped fresh parsley
    Pinch cayenne pepper

Heat the butter in a large pot over medium heat. Add the onions and sauté, stirring, until golden brown, about 15 minutes. Add the garlic and sauté until garlic is softened, about 3 minutes more.

Cut about half of the button mushrooms into slivers and set aside. Add the cremini, portobello, and remaining button mushrooms to the onion mixture and sauté for 5 minutes, or until the mushrooms are golden. Add enough stock to barely cover the mushroom mixture, then add the evaporated milk. Bring to a simmer, reduce the heat to low, cover partially, and cook until the mushrooms are softened, about 20 minutes. Transfer the soup to a blender and puree. Return the soup to the pot, add the reserved mushroom slivers and salt and pepper to taste. Stir in the parsley and cayenne and reheat briefly. Serve hot.

Curried Cauliflower Soup

SERVES 5 OR 6

This great soup, another creation of our friend Carol Bronz, the "soup nurse," has a little kick of curry.

4 **tablespoons (½ stick) butter**
3 **medium onions, sliced**
2 **medium heads cauliflower (about 2 pounds total), broken into florets**
4 **cups homemade chicken stock (page 58)**
1½ **teaspoons curry powder**
   Salt and freshly ground pepper

Heat the butter in a large pot over medium heat. Add the onions, and sauté, stirring, until golden, about 15 minutes.

Add about three-fourths of the cauliflower florets and the stock to the pot. Bring to a boil, cover, reduce the heat to low, and simmer until the cauliflower is very soft, about 20 minutes.

Transfer the cauliflower mixture to a blender and puree. Return the puree to the pot and add the remaining cauliflower florets, the curry powder, and salt and pepper to taste. Increase the heat to medium and simmer until the cauliflower is soft, about 10 minutes. Serve hot.

Curried Broccoli-Potato Soup

SERVES 8

This rich soup is creamy without containing any cream.
It's excellent hot or cold.

1½   tablespoons butter
1   cup chopped shallots (about 8)
2   large garlic cloves, minced
4   cups homemade chicken stock (page 58)
1   teaspoon curry powder, or more to taste
⅛   teaspoon freshly ground pepper
1   bunch broccoli (about 1¼ pounds), separated
      into florets, stems cut into ½-inch cubes
2   medium potatoes, peeled and cut
      into ½-inch cubes
2   cups 1% milk
    Salt

Heat the butter in a large pot over medium heat. Add the shallots
and garlic and sauté, stirring, until soft, about 5 minutes. Add the
stock, curry powder, and pepper and bring to a boil.

Add the broccoli and potatoes to the pot. Return to a boil, reduce
the heat to low, cover, and simmer for 20 minutes, or until the vegetables are tender. With a slotted spoon, transfer about half of the broccoli to a medium bowl and set aside.

Transfer the soup to a blender and puree in batches. Return the
soup to the pot, add the reserved broccoli and the milk, and reheat over
low heat. Season with salt to taste and serve hot.

New England Clam Chowder

SERVES 6

The son of our friend Julie Eckhert loved the chowder served at the Maritime Center in Norwalk, Connecticut, so she experimented at home until she got it just right. A word of caution, however, about the clams and juice: Bottled clam juice and canned clams frequently contain MSG, a common headache trigger. At least one brand is specifically labeled "no MSG." That's what you should choose.

8 tablespoons (1 stick) butter
3 medium potatoes, peeled and diced
1½ cups chopped carrots (about 4 medium)
1 large onion, chopped
4 8-ounce bottles no-MSG clam juice
1½ cups 1% milk
1 6½-ounce can no-MSG chopped clams
1 bay leaf
¾ teaspoon dried thyme, crumbled
¾ teaspoon dried dill, crumbled
¼ cup all-purpose flour
¼ teaspoon ground nutmeg
Salt and freshly ground pepper

Heat the butter in a large pot over medium heat. Add the potatoes, carrots, and onion and sauté, stirring, until the onion is soft, about 5 minutes. Add the clam juice, increase the heat to high, and bring to a boil. Reduce the heat to low, cover partially, and simmer until the potatoes are soft, about 20 minutes. Add 1 cup of the milk, the clams and their juice, the bay leaf, thyme, and dill. Increase the heat to high and bring to a boil. Whisk the flour with the remaining ½ cup milk in a small bowl until smooth. Whisk the flour mixture gradually into the soup until combined. Add the nutmeg and salt and pepper to taste. Simmer for 5 minutes more to blend the flavors. Serve hot.

Pasta

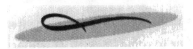

Roasted Garlic Linguine

SERVES 2 AS A MAIN COURSE, 4 AS AN APPETIZER

David loved eating this dish at Italian restaurants so much that he begged me to come up with a headache-free version. Here it is . . . and he says it's better than the restaurant dish.

⅓	cup canola oil
1½	tablespoons butter
8–10	garlic cloves, crushed with the flat side of a knife
8	ounces dried linguine
	Salt
	Freshly ground pepper

Heat the oil and butter in a small skillet over low heat. Add the garlic and sauté, stirring often, until slightly browned, about 10 minutes.

Meanwhile, cook the linguine in a large pot of boiling, salted water until al dente, about 8 minutes. Drain the linguine and transfer it to a large serving bowl. Toss the linguine with the garlic mixture, season with salt and pepper to taste, and serve.

Farfalle with Tomato-Basil Sauce

SERVES 2

Because of the limits on tomatoes on the headache-prevention
diet, this is about as close as a headache sufferer
can get to pasta with red sauce. If you eat more than one serving,
you risk exceeding the limit on tomatoes.

- 2 **tablespoons canola oil**
- 1 **tablespoon butter**
- ⅔ **cup chopped tomato (about 1 medium tomato)**
- ⅓ **cup chopped fresh basil**
- ¼ **cup skim milk**
- 1 **teaspoon fresh lemon juice**
- 8 **ounces dried farfalle**
  Salt and freshly ground pepper

Heat the oil and butter in a large skillet over medium heat. Add the
tomato and basil and sauté, stirring occasionally, for about 5 minutes,
or until the oil mixture turns slightly pink. Add the milk and lemon
juice, reduce the heat to medium, and simmer, stirring frequently, for
5 minutes, or until hot and well blended.

Meanwhile, cook the farfalle in a large pot of boiling, salted water
until al dente, 10 to 12 minutes. Drain the farfalle and transfer it to a
large serving bowl. Toss the farfalle with the tomato-basil sauce, season
with salt and pepper to taste, and serve.

Orzo with Spinach, Tomato, and Ricotta Cheese

SERVES 2 AS A MAIN COURSE,
4 AS AN APPETIZER OR SIDE DISH

When you taste this pasta, you won't miss the aged cheeses that are usually added. Ricotta and a modest amount of tomato give the dish an authentic Italian flavor.

8	**ounces dried orzo**
1	**teaspoon canola oil**
½	**medium onion, chopped**
3	**garlic cloves, thinly sliced**
10–12	**ounces fresh spinach, cleaned and chopped**
1	**cup chopped fresh tomato**
¾	**cup part skim-milk ricotta cheese**
¾	**teaspoon dried oregano, crumbled**
	Salt
⅛	**teaspoon freshly ground pepper**

Cook the orzo in a large pot of boiling, salted water until it is soft, 9 to 10 minutes. Drain the orzo and transfer it to a large serving bowl, cover, and keep warm.

Meanwhile, heat the oil in a large skillet over medium heat. Add the onion and garlic and sauté, stirring occasionally, for 5 minutes, or until softened. Add the spinach and tomato and sauté, stirring, until the spinach is wilted, about 3 minutes more. Stir in the ricotta cheese, oregano, ½ teaspoon salt, and the pepper. Add to the orzo, toss thoroughly, and serve.

Farfalle
with Wild Mushrooms

SERVES 4

This pasta dish is extraordinarily flavorful without relying
on the usual tomato sauce or cheese.

2 **tablespoons (¼ stick) butter**
2 **tablespoons canola oil**
3 **tablespoons finely chopped shallots**
12 **ounces assorted fresh wild mushrooms (cremini,**
   portobello, chanterelle, shiitake, oyster), sliced
1 **cup homemade chicken stock (page 58)**
2 **tablespoons tomato paste**
1 **pound dried farfalle**
   Salt and freshly ground pepper

Heat the butter and oil in a large skillet over medium heat. Add the
shallots and sauté, stirring, for 4 minutes, or until translucent. Add the
mushrooms and sauté, stirring, for 6 minutes more, or until they are
tender. Add the stock and cook until most of the liquid has evaporated,
about 10 minutes. Add the tomato paste and mix thoroughly. Remove
from the heat, cover, and keep warm.

Meanwhile, cook the farfalle in a large pot of boiling, salted water
until al dente, 10 to 12 minutes. Drain the farfalle and transfer it to a
large bowl. Add the mushroom mixture, season with salt and pepper to
taste, toss, and serve.

Penne with Vegetables and Garlic

SERVES 4

In order for the different vegetables in this pasta dish
to be cooked evenly, they must be stir-fried individually and
then tossed with the pasta. The oil in which the vegetables are
cooked takes on their flavors and becomes the sauce.

6 **tablespoons canola oil**
1 **pound carrots, peeled and cut into 1½-to-2-inch
    diagonal slices**
1 **pound pencil-thin asparagus spears, ends snapped
    off, cut into 2-inch pieces**
1 **pound white button mushrooms, thinly sliced**
4 **garlic cloves, cut into slivers, plus 1 tablespoon
    minced garlic**
1 **pound dried penne**
   Salt

Heat 1 tablespoon of the oil in a large skillet over medium heat.
Add the carrots and stir-fry until just tender, about 10 minutes. With
a slotted spoon, transfer the carrots to a platter. Heat 1 tablespoon
more oil in the skillet, add the asparagus, and stir-fry until bright green
and crisp-tender, about 4 minutes. Transfer the asparagus to the platter. Heat 1 tablespoon more oil in the skillet, add the mushrooms, and
stir-fry until golden, about 5 minutes. Transfer the mushrooms to the

platter. Heat 1 tablespoon more oil in the skillet, add the slivered garlic, and stir-fry until it just begins to color, about 5 minutes. Transfer the garlic to the platter. Heat the remaining 2 tablespoons oil in the skillet, add the minced garlic, and stir-fry until it begins to color, about 4 minutes. Return all the vegetables to the skillet and toss to mix.

Meanwhile, cook the penne in a large pot of boiling, salted water until al dente, 10 to 12 minutes. Drain the penne and transfer it to a large serving bowl. Add the vegetable mixture, add salt to taste, toss together, and serve.

Garden Capellini

SERVES 4

This light pasta may be eaten warm or cold.
Fresh mint provides a refreshing accent.

½ **cup dry-packed sun-dried tomatoes**
1 **pound dried capellini**
2 **tablespoons (¼ stick) butter**
¾ **pound white button mushrooms, sliced**
1 **pound asparagus spears, ends snapped off,
    halved crosswise**
1 **cup green peas**
¼ **cup canola oil**
¼ **cup chopped fresh parsley**
2 **tablespoons chopped fresh mint**
1 **tablespoon fresh lime juice**
    Salt
    Freshly ground pepper

Lime slices or fresh mint sprig for garnish

Blanch the sun-dried tomatoes in a small pot of boiling water until softened, about 10 minutes; drain. Cut into thin strips and set aside.

Meanwhile, cook the capellini in a large pot of boiling, salted water until al dente, 4 to 6 minutes. Drain the capellini and set aside.

Melt the butter in a large saucepan over medium heat. Add the mushrooms and sauté, stirring, for 4 minutes, or until softened. Add the asparagus, peas, and sun-dried tomatoes and sauté for 4 minutes more, stirring occasionally. Mix in the capellini and oil and sauté for 2 to 3 minutes, or until heated through. Add the parsley and mint and stir until combined. Add the lime juice and salt and pepper to taste. Toss again and serve warm or cold, garnished with the lime slices or mint.

Rigatoni with Eggplant

SERVES 4

This recipe is courtesy of Michelle Cirino, the head receptionist at Laura's office. Her family absolutely loves this dish. So does ours.

1	cup fresh bread crumbs
¼	cup chopped fresh parsley
½	teaspoon chopped fresh basil or ¼ teaspoon dried, crumbled
	Salt
¼	teaspoon freshly ground pepper
1	large eggplant, peeled and cut into 1-inch-wide, ½-inch-thick strips
	All-purpose flour
2	large eggs, lightly beaten
5–6	tablespoons canola oil
2	medium tomatoes, chopped
1	medium onion, chopped
1½	cups homemade chicken stock (page 58)
½	teaspoon chopped fresh oregano or ¼ teaspoon dried, crumbled
	Pinch crushed red pepper flakes
1	pound dried rigatoni

Combine the bread crumbs, parsley, basil, ½ teaspoon salt, and pepper in a large, shallow bowl. Coat the eggplant strips on both sides with the flour, then with the egg, then with the bread-crumb mixture.

Heat 1 tablespoon oil in a large skillet over medium heat. Fry the eggplant strips in batches, turning, until they are golden brown and tender when pierced with a fork, adding 1 tablespoon oil for each batch of eggplant. Drain the eggplant strips on paper towels.

Wipe out the skillet. Add 1 tablespoon oil and sauté the tomatoes and onion, stirring, until the onion is soft, about 5 minutes. Add the stock, oregano and red pepper flakes and bring to a simmer.

Meanwhile, cook the rigatoni in a large pot of boiling, salted water until al dente, 10 to 12 minutes. Drain the rigatoni and transfer it to a large bowl. Add the tomato sauce and toss well. Arrange the eggplant strips on top of the pasta and serve.

Linguine
with White Clam Sauce

SERVES 2

This traditional Italian favorite has two headache hurdles that are easy to overcome. Substitute canola oil for olive oil, and be sure to buy clam juice and canned clams without MSG. The taste is primo!

2 6½-ounce cans no-MSG minced clams
1 8-ounce bottle no-MSG clam juice
3 tablespoons butter
1 tablespoon canola oil
2 garlic cloves, thinly sliced
2 teaspoons all-purpose flour
¼ cup chopped fresh parsley, plus a few
    sprigs fresh parsley for garnish
1 teaspoon dried thyme, crumbled
8 ounces dried linguine
    Salt

Drain the clams and set them aside, pouring the juices into a large glass measuring cup. Add enough of the bottled clam juice to measure 1½ cups.

Heat 2 tablespoons of the butter and the oil in a medium skillet over low heat. Add the garlic and sauté, pressing down on the garlic with a wooden spoon to release the flavor, until the garlic is golden. (If you're a garlic lover, leave it in the skillet. If not, discard it.)

Sprinkle the flour into the skillet and cook, stirring constantly, for 1 minute. Slowly stir in the clam juice. Add the parsley and thyme, increase the heat to high, and bring to a boil. Reduce the heat to low and simmer, stirring frequently, for 8 minutes, or until slightly thickened.

Meanwhile, cook the linguine in a large pot of boiling, salted water until al dente, about 8 minutes. Drain the linguine and return it to the pot. Add the remaining 1 tablespoon butter and toss well.

Just before serving, add the clams to the sauce in the skillet, add salt to taste, and cook just until heated through. Pour the sauce over the linguine and serve immediately, garnished with the parsley sprigs.

Rotini with Chicken and Sun-Dried Tomatoes

SERVES 4

In winter, when fresh tomatoes are not at their peak,
this pasta dish brings back a hint of summer.

⅔ **cup dry-packed sun-dried tomatoes**
1 **tablespoon canola oil**
1 **tablespoon butter**
6 **garlic cloves, minced**
  All-purpose flour
1 **pound boneless, skinless chicken breasts, cut into**
    1-inch-wide strips
⅓ **cup chopped fresh basil**
1¼ **cups homemade chicken stock (page 58)**
1 **pound dried rotini**
  Salt and freshly ground pepper

Preheat the oven to 200 degrees F.

Blanch the sun-dried tomatoes in a small pot of boiling water until softened, about 10 minutes; drain. Cut into thin strips and set aside.

Heat the oil and butter in a large skillet over medium heat. Add the garlic and sauté until soft, 3 to 4 minutes.

Place the flour on a large plate and dredge the chicken strips. Add the chicken to the skillet and sauté, stirring, until no longer pink, about 8 minutes. Add the sun-dried tomatoes and basil and sauté, stirring, for 5 minutes, or until heated through.

Transfer the chicken mixture to a 13-x-9-inch baking dish and keep warm in the oven. Reduce the heat to medium, add the stock to the skillet, and cook, stirring, scraping up the browned bits from the bottom, until the broth is syrupy.

Meanwhile, cook the rotini in a large pot of boiling, salted water until al dente, 10 to 12 minutes. Drain.

Add the rotini and stock mixture to the baking dish, toss well, add salt and pepper to taste, and serve.

Chicken, Turkey, and Duck

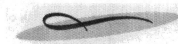

Chicken-Asparagus Salad

SERVES 4

This salad is fit for a meal. The raspberry vinegar gives it a wonderful taste and is usually not a problem for headache sufferers. It's a great treat with the first asparagus of the season.

6 **tablespoons canola oil**
1 **pound boneless, skinless chicken breasts, cut into ¾-inch-wide strips**
   Salt and freshly ground pepper
1 **pound asparagus spears, ends snapped off, halved crosswise**
2 **tablespoons raspberry vinegar**
1½ **teaspoons fresh lemon juice**
½ **teaspoon dry mustard**
¼ **teaspoon dried tarragon, crumbled**
2 **heads Boston lettuce, cleaned and torn into bite-size pieces**
20–25 **fresh raspberries (optional)**

Heat the oil in a medium skillet over medium heat. Add the chicken and sauté, stirring, until cooked through, about 5 minutes. Season with salt and pepper to taste, transfer to a plate, and set aside. Reserve the oil in the skillet.

Meanwhile, cook the asparagus in a large saucepan of boiling water until crisp-tender, about 3 minutes. Drain the asparagus and rinse it with cold water. Drain again and set aside.

Whisk together the reserved oil, the vinegar, lemon juice, mustard and tarragon in a small bowl.

Place the lettuce, chicken, and asparagus on a platter, add the dressing and toss gently. Garnish with raspberries, if desired, and serve.

Lemon-Glazed Chicken

SERVES 4

This no-fuss chicken dish has an agreeable tangy sweetness
that is different from the usual lemon chicken.

GLAZE

- ⅓ **cup light corn syrup**
- 2 **tablespoons apple juice**
- ½ **tablespoon finely grated lemon rind**
- 1 **tablespoon fresh lemon juice**
- ¼ **teaspoon salt**

- 4 **boneless, skinless chicken breasts**
  (about 1½ pounds total)
- 1 **tablespoon canola oil**
- 1 **teaspoon salt**
- ¼ **teaspoon freshly ground pepper**

Preheat the oven to 350 degrees F.

GLAZE: Combine the corn syrup, apple juice, lemon rind,
lemon juice, and salt in a small bowl.

Place the chicken in a 13-x-9-inch baking dish. Brush the oil over
the chicken and sprinkle with the salt and pepper. Brush some of the
glaze over the chicken. Bake for 20 to 30 minutes, brushing frequently
ly with the glaze, or until the chicken is golden brown and the juices
run clear when it is pierced with a fork. Serve hot.

Garlic Chicken

SERVES 4

Here's a quick and easy dinner with a lot of flavor.
If you're a garlic lover, you'll definitely love this one!

1   **whole garlic head**
4   **boneless, skinless chicken breasts**
      (about 1½ pounds total)
      About 1½ tablespoons canola oil
½   **teaspoon salt**
¼   **teaspoon freshly ground pepper**

Preheat the oven to 375 degrees F.

Separate the garlic into cloves. Peel the cloves and use the flat side of a knife to smash them lightly.

Place the chicken in a 13-x-9-inch baking dish, brush with the oil, and sprinkle with the salt and pepper. Place the garlic cloves on top of the chicken.

Cover the dish with aluminum foil and bake for 20 minutes. Uncover and bake for 10 minutes more, or until the juices run clear when the chicken is pierced with a fork. Serve hot.

Orange Chicken

SERVES 4

Although citrus fruits are limited in the headache-prevention diet, there is enough orange in this dish to give the chicken plenty of zip.

2   **large navel oranges**
½   **cup all-purpose flour**
    Salt and freshly ground pepper
4   **boneless, skinless chicken breasts (about**
      1½ pounds total), pounded to ½ inch thick
1   **tablespoon butter**
1   **tablespoon canola oil**
¼   **cup orange juice**
¾   **cup homemade chicken stock (page 58)**
1½   **teaspoons orange marmalade**

Peel the oranges, being careful to remove all the white membrane around the outside. Using a sharp knife, separate the oranges into sections, cutting between the membranes. Discard the membranes. Set orange sections aside.

Place the flour in a large, shallow dish and season with salt and pepper to taste. Dredge the chicken in the flour.

Heat the butter and oil in a large skillet over medium heat. Add the chicken and sauté in batches if necessary, turning, until golden brown, about 8 minutes per side. Transfer to a serving platter, set aside, and keep warm.

Add the orange juice to the skillet and cook, stirring, scraping up the browned bits from the bottom. Add the stock and cook until the sauce becomes syrupy, about 8 minutes. Add the marmalade and stir until it dissolves. Remove from the heat and stir in the orange sections. Pour the sauce over the chicken and serve.

Chicken and Mushrooms in Cream Sauce

SERVES 4

This dinner looks delicate but tastes hearty.
It's great with mashed potatoes.

3   **tablespoons butter**
2   **tablespoons canola oil**
1   **pound white button mushrooms,**
      stems trimmed, sliced
⅓   **cup plus 1 tablespoon all-purpose flour**
      Salt and freshly ground pepper
4   **boneless, skinless chicken breasts (about**
      1½ pounds total), cut into 1-inch cubes
1   **cup homemade chicken stock (page 58)**
½   **cup evaporated skim milk, heated**

Heat 1 tablespoon of the butter and 1 tablespoon of the oil in a large skillet over medium heat. Add the mushrooms and sauté, stirring occasionally, for 5 minutes, or until softened. Transfer to a medium bowl and set aside.

Place the ⅓ cup flour in a large, shallow dish and season with salt and pepper to taste. Dredge the chicken in the flour. Add 1 tablespoon of the butter and the remaining 1 tablespoon oil to the skillet. Add the chicken and sauté, stirring, until lightly browned, about 10 minutes. Transfer the chicken to the bowl with the mushrooms and set aside.

Reduce the heat to medium, add the stock to the skillet, and cook, stirring, scraping up the browned bits from the bottom. Reduce the heat to low and slowly whisk in the evaporated milk. If you want a thicker sauce, work the remaining 1 tablespoon butter and the 1 table-spoon flour into a paste in a small bowl, increase the heat to medium, and whisk into the sauce a little at a time, until the sauce reaches the desired thickness.

Add the reserved chicken and mushrooms to the skillet and cook for 5 minutes, or until heated through. Serve hot.

Chicken with Artichoke Hearts

SERVES 4

Serve this lemony chicken dish over white rice or with bread to sop up the sauce.

2   **large eggs**
⅓   **cup plus ½ tablespoon all-purpose flour**
4   **boneless, skinless chicken breasts (about 1½ pounds total)**
2   **tablespoons canola oil**
1½ **tablespoons butter**
1   **pound white button mushrooms, stems trimmed, sliced**
1   **14-ounce can water-packed artichoke hearts, drained and quartered**
1   **cup homemade chicken stock (page 58)**
2   **tablespoons fresh lemon juice**
    Salt and freshly ground pepper

Lightly beat the eggs in a large, shallow bowl and place the ⅓ cup flour in a separate large, shallow bowl. Coat the chicken with the egg, then dredge in the flour.

Heat 1 tablespoon of the oil and 1 tablespoon of the butter in a large skillet over medium heat. Add the chicken and sauté, in batches if necessary, turning until lightly browned on both sides, about 5 minutes per side. Place the chicken in a 13-x-9-inch baking dish. Set the skillet with the drippings aside.

Preheat the oven to 350 degrees F.

Heat the remaining 1 tablespoon oil in a separate large skillet over medium heat. Add the mushrooms and sauté, stirring occasionally, for 3 to 4 minutes, or until softened. Add the artichokes and cook for 5 minutes more, or until heated through. Transfer the mushrooms and artichokes to the baking dish with the chicken.

Place the skillet with the chicken drippings over medium heat. Add the stock and bring to a boil, scraping up the browned bits from the bottom.

Meanwhile, work the remaining ½ tablespoon butter and the ½ tablespoon flour into a paste in a small bowl. Whisk into the stock mixture a little at a time until the stock is thickened. Whisk in the lemon juice and season with salt and pepper to taste. Pour the sauce over the chicken mixture and cover the baking dish with aluminum foil.

Bake for 20 minutes, or until the juices run clear when the chicken is pierced with a fork. Serve immediately.

Herbed Roast Chicken with Mushroom Gravy

SERVES 4

This dish is a favorite on Rosh Hashanah, the Jewish New Year. The herbs provide a flavorful crust, transforming an ordinary roast chicken into a special-occasion dinner.

CHICKEN

1   3-to-4-pound roasting chicken
1   tablespoon chopped fresh rosemary
       or 1 teaspoon dried, crumbled
1   tablespoon chopped fresh thyme
       or 1 teaspoon dried, crumbled
1   tablespoon chopped fresh tarragon
       or 1 teaspoon dried, crumbled
½   teaspoon salt
½   teaspoon freshly ground pepper
1½ teaspoons canola oil
1   tablespoon butter, melted
½   cup homemade chicken stock (page 58)

GRAVY

2   tablespoons butter
8   ounces portobello mushrooms,
       stems trimmed, sliced
    Pinch dried rosemary, crumbled
¼   cup all-purpose flour
2   cups homemade chicken stock (page 58)
    Salt

Preheat the oven to 450 degrees F.

CHICKEN: Rinse the chicken inside and out with cold water and pat it dry with paper towels. In a small bowl, combine the rosemary, thyme, tarragon, salt, and pepper. Brush the chicken with the oil, then rub the herb mixture over the chicken and place it in a shallow roasting pan. Drizzle the melted butter over the chicken.

Pour the ½ cup stock into the roasting pan. Cover the chicken loosely with aluminum foil and roast for 20 minutes. Reduce the oven temperature to 350 degrees F. Remove the foil and roast the chicken 20 to 40 minutes, basting once or twice with the pan juices, until the juices run clear when the thickest part of a thigh is pierced with a fork. Transfer the chicken to a cutting board and let stand for 10 minutes before carving. Reserve the pan juices.

GRAVY: Meanwhile, melt the butter in a large skillet over medium heat. Add the mushrooms and sauté, stirring, until golden, about 10 minutes. Reduce the heat to low, add the rosemary, and cook until hot and well blended.

Place the flour in a medium bowl. Whisk in the pan juices a little at a time to form a paste. Stir the flour mixture into the mushrooms, then add the 2 cups stock and stir over low heat until the gravy is thickened and smooth. Season with salt to taste. Carve the chicken and serve with the gravy.

Mexican Chicken

SERVES 4

This headache-safe marinade produces chicken
with a great south-of-the-border taste.

⅓ **cup plus 1½ tablespoons canola oil**
3 **garlic cloves, minced**
5 **teaspoons fresh lime juice**
1 **tablespoon chopped fresh cilantro**
½ **teaspoon ground cumin**
¼ **teaspoon chili powder**
2 **pounds boneless, skinless chicken breasts, cut into**
    1½-inch-wide strips

Combine the ⅓ cup oil, the garlic, lime juice, cilantro, cumin, and chili powder in a 13-x-9-inch baking dish. Add the chicken, toss to coat, cover, and marinate in the refrigerator for at least 2 hours or overnight.

Heat the 1½ tablespoons oil in a large skillet over medium-high heat. Add the chicken and sauté, stirring, until cooked through, about 10 minutes. Serve hot.

Cornish Hens and Wild Rice with Apricot Sauce

SERVES 4

This recipe has been in the family of our friend Julie Eckhert for years, but it called for a generous amount of orange liqueur, which can cause headaches. Julie experimented with different ingredients to replace the flavor of the liqueur . . . and her child likes this version better than the original!

1	**15-ounce can apricot halves in heavy syrup, drained, 2 tablespoons syrup reserved**
1	**rounded tablespoon apricot preserves**
1	**tablespoon dry mustard, dissolved in 1 teaspoon water**
1	**cup wild rice**
1½	**teaspoons butter**
1	**cup chopped celery**
3	**scallions, chopped**
2	**1-to-1½-pound Cornish hens**
¼	**teaspoon salt**

Place the apricots, the reserved syrup, preserves, and mustard mixture in a blender and blend until smooth. Pour the apricot sauce into a small saucepan.

Cook the wild rice according to the package directions, about 45 minutes.

Meanwhile, heat the butter in a large skillet over medium heat. Add the celery and scallions and sauté, stirring occasionally, until soft, about 3 minutes. When the rice is done, stir in the celery mixture, cover, and keep warm.

Meanwhile, preheat the broiler. Rinse the Cornish hens inside and out with cold water and pat them dry with paper towels. Cut the hens in half through the breastbone so that each half contains a leg. Place the hen halves on a broiler pan skin side down and broil about 4 inches from the heat for 10 minutes. Turn the hens and broil for 10 minutes more. Remove the hens from the oven, cool slightly, then remove as much of the skin as possible.

Preheat the oven to 400 degrees F.

Sprinkle the hens with ⅛ teaspoon of the salt and brush them with some of the apricot sauce. Bake for 10 minutes. Sprinkle the hens with the remaining ⅛ teaspoon salt and brush with more apricot sauce. Turn and bake for 10 minutes, or until the juices run clear when the thickest part of a thigh is pierced with a fork.

Heat the remaining apricot sauce over low heat. Spoon some of the rice onto each plate, top each serving of rice with a hen half, spoon some of the apricot sauce over the hens, and serve.

Cranberry-Glazed Turkey Breast

SERVES 6

This is a fast, convenient twist on traditional turkey and cranberry sauce. The cranberry glaze produces a flavorful and moist turkey breast.

1	**4-to-6-pound bone-in turkey breast**
1½	**tablespoons canola oil**
¾	**teaspoon salt**
½	**teaspoon garlic powder**
¼	**teaspoon freshly ground pepper**
1	**16-ounce can whole-berry cranberry sauce**
¼	**cup homemade chicken stock (page 58)**
¼	**cup apple juice**

Preheat the oven to 450 degrees F.

Rub the turkey breast all over with the oil and season with the salt, garlic powder, and pepper. Place the turkey in a shallow roasting pan. Reduce the oven temperature to 325 degrees F and roast the turkey breast for 20 minutes per pound, or until a meat thermometer registers 170 degrees F, basting occasionally with the pan juices.

Meanwhile, place the cranberry sauce, stock, and apple juice in a small saucepan over low heat and cook, stirring occasionally, until the cranberry sauce melts.

About 30 minutes before the turkey breast is done, brush it all over with the cranberry glaze, then pour the remaining glaze over it. Baste with the pan juices every 5 minutes until the turkey breast is done. Let the turkey breast rest for 10 minutes. Carve into thin slices and serve with the pan juices on the side.

Braised Turkey Breast with Dried Cherry–Orange Sauce

SERVES 6

Laura's mom serves this dish at family dinners.
Make sure the dried cherries do not contain
headache-triggering preservatives, such as sulfur.

1   **3-pound boneless turkey breast**
    Salt and freshly ground pepper
5   **tablespoons butter, at room temperature**
2   **tablespoons peeled and minced fresh ginger**
2   **large garlic cloves, minced**
1   **tablespoon chopped fresh cilantro**
1   **tablespoon canola oil**
2   **cups orange juice**
1   **cup preservative-free dried cherries**
1   **bay leaf**
    Finely grated rind of 1 orange

Preheat the oven to 325 degrees F.

Place the turkey breast skin side down on a work surface. Season the side facing up with salt and pepper to taste.

Combine 3 tablespoons of the butter, 1 tablespoon of the ginger, 1 of the minced garlic cloves, and the cilantro in a small bowl. Mash into a paste with a fork. Spread the paste over the turkey breast. Roll the turkey breast into a roast and tie it with kitchen twine. Rub the outside of the turkey breast with 1 tablespoon of the butter and season with salt and pepper to taste.

Heat the remaining 1 tablespoon butter and the oil in a large Dutch oven over medium heat. Add the remaining 1 tablespoon ginger and the remaining 1 minced garlic clove and sauté for 1 minute, or until slightly softened. Place the turkey breast in the Dutch oven and add the orange juice, dried cherries, and bay leaf. Increase the heat to high and bring to a simmer, then cover the Dutch oven and place it in the oven. Bake for 1¼ to 1½ hours, basting occasionally, or until a meat thermometer inserted into the center of the turkey breast registers 170 degrees F.

Remove the Dutch oven from the oven and let stand, covered, for 15 minutes. Transfer the turkey breast to a cutting board.

Place the Dutch oven over high heat and add the orange rind. Simmer for about 5 minutes, or until the sauce is reduced by half. Remove the bay leaf. Season with salt and pepper to taste.

Slice the turkey breast and place on a serving platter. Spoon the sauce over the turkey and serve.

Duck à l'Orange with Apple Stuffing

SERVES 2

Crisp-skinned duck topped with a not-too-sweet orange sauce and served with an apple stuffing sounds like a restaurant specialty, but it's not difficult to prepare at home, and it's well worth the effort.

DUCK

1 4-pound duck
   Salt and freshly ground pepper
2 tablespoons butter, melted

APPLE STUFFING

8 slices whole wheat bread, cut into 2-inch cubes
1 cup homemade chicken stock (page 58)
3 tablespoons butter
⅓ cup chopped onion
⅓ cup chopped celery
½ cup peeled, thinly sliced apple
2 teaspoons dried sage, crumbled
2 teaspoons no-MSG poultry seasoning
½ teaspoon salt
   Freshly ground pepper

ORANGE SAUCE

⅓ cup orange marmalade
⅓ cup orange juice
6 cloves
1 cinnamon stick

2   teaspoons cornstarch
¼   cup cold water

1   orange, sliced, for garnish
4   sprigs fresh parsley for garnish

D U C K : Place a shallow roasting pan in the oven and preheat the oven to 350 degrees F.

Sprinkle the duck with salt and pepper to taste and brush it with the melted butter. Place the duck breast side up in the preheated roasting pan and roast for 1 hour. Remove the pan from the oven and drain off and discard the pan juices. Increase the oven temperature to 450 degrees F. Turn the duck over and roast for 15 minutes more. Remove the pan from the oven and drain off and discard the pan juices. Turn the duck again and roast for 15 minutes more. Remove the duck from the oven, drain off and discard the pan juices and let cool completely (refrigerate it until the next day, if you wish). Split the duck in half lengthwise.

A P P L E   S T U F F I N G : Place the bread cubes in a medium bowl and pour the stock over them. Heat the butter in a large skillet over medium heat. Add the onion and celery and sauté, stirring occasionally, until they are soft, about 10 minutes. Remove from the heat. Drain the bread cubes and add them to the skillet, mixing thoroughly. Add the apple, sage, poultry seasoning, salt, and pepper to taste and mix well.

Preheat the oven to 350 degrees F.

Place the stuffing in two mounds in the roasting pan and place a duck half on each mound. Roast the duck for 15 minutes, or until the skin is crisp.

O R A N G E   S A U C E : Meanwhile, combine the marmalade, orange juice, cloves, and cinnamon stick in a small saucepan over medium heat. Bring to a boil. Dissolve the cornstarch in the cold water and stir it into the orange mixture. Reduce the heat to low and simmer until the sauce is thickened and clear. Remove the cloves and cinnamon stick.

Place a duck half with stuffing on each serving plate. Cover with the orange sauce and garnish with the orange and parsley.

Beef, Pork, Lamb, and Veal

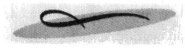

Individual Meat Loaves with Mustard Butter

SERVES 6

David loves mustard. Since he shouldn't eat store-bought mustard, Laura's mom invented this headache-safe alternative.

MEAT LOAVES

2 **pounds lean ground beef**
2 **large eggs**
⅓ **cup dry bread crumbs**
⅓ **cup finely chopped celery**
⅓ **cup finely grated carrots**
1 **teaspoon salt**
1 **teaspoon dry mustard**
½ **teaspoon garlic powder**
¼ **teaspoon freshly ground pepper**

MUSTARD BUTTER

4 **tablespoons (½ stick) butter, at room temperature**
1½ **teaspoons dry mustard**
½ **teaspoon dried tarragon, crumbled**
¼ **teaspoon fresh lemon juice**

MEAT LOAVES: Preheat the oven to 350 degrees F.

With wet hands, mix together all the ingredients in a large bowl. Form the meat mixture into 6 loaves, about 4 inches long and 2½ inches wide.

Place the meat loaves in a roasting pan. Add ¼ cup water to the pan and bake the meat loaves for 50 minutes, or until brown and crisp, basting occasionally with the pan juices and adding more water if necessary.

MUSTARD BUTTER: Meanwhile, combine the butter, mustard, tarragon, and lemon juice in a small bowl. Let stand in the refrigerator for 30 minutes.

Top each meat loaf with 2 teaspoons of the mustard butter and serve immediately.

Asian Ginger Beef with Broccoli

SERVES 4

Chinese food was one of the things David missed most when he began the headache-prevention diet, so I came up with this recipe. It's a great Chinese-style dish without soy sauce or MSG. Serve with rice.

- **2 tablespoons canola oil**
- **2–3 garlic cloves, minced**
- **2 teaspoons peeled and grated fresh ginger**
- **1 pound tender, lean beef (such as sirloin), cut into ½-inch-wide strips**
- **1 pound broccoli, cut into bite-size pieces**
- **1 cup canned baby corn, halved crosswise**
- **1 teaspoon sugar**
- **1 teaspoon salt**
- **1 teaspoon fresh lemon juice**

Heat the oil in a large skillet over medium heat. Add the garlic and ginger and sauté, stirring occasionally, until softened, about 5 minutes. Add the beef and sauté, stirring frequently, until browned, about 5 minutes. Add the broccoli, corn, sugar, salt, and lemon juice and sauté, stirring frequently, until the broccoli is crisp-tender, about 10 minutes. Serve.

Steak au Poivre

SERVES 4

This special dish is usually made with a cream sauce and flamed with brandy. But even the most discerning taste buds will be fooled by the evaporated skim milk, and you won't miss the alcohol.

> 2   tablespoons black peppercorns
> 4   8-ounce filet mignon steaks
>   Salt
>   Canola oil
> 4   tablespoons (½ stick) butter
> 2   tablespoons finely chopped shallots
> 1½   cups evaporated skim milk
> 1   teaspoon dry mustard

Preheat the oven to 300 degrees F.

Using a rolling pin, coarsely crush the peppercorns. Coat the steaks with the pepper on both sides, pressing the pepper into the meat with your hands. Season with salt to taste.

Lightly coat the bottom of a large, heavy skillet with oil and place over medium-high heat. Add the steaks 2 at a time and cook, turning once, to the desired doneness, about 5 minutes for rare, 7 minutes for medium-rare and 9 minutes for medium. Repeat with the remaining 2 steaks. Keep the steaks warm on an ovenproof plate in the oven.

Add the butter and shallots to the skillet and sauté over medium heat, stirring, for about 3 minutes, or until soft but not browned. Add the evaporated milk and simmer for 10 minutes, stirring frequently, until thick enough to coat the back of a spoon. Remove from the heat and stir in the mustard. Pour over the steaks and serve immediately.

Braised Barbecue Beef

SERVES 6

This beef has the flavor of a real down-home barbecue,
but when you taste it, you won't believe it's made in the oven.
Begin preparing this dish the day before you plan to serve it.

1   **tablespoon dry mustard**
1   **tablespoon paprika**
1   **teaspoon salt**
½   **teaspoon freshly ground pepper**
1   **4½-to-5-pound beef brisket**
¼   **cup canola oil**
1   **cup cider vinegar**
⅔   **cup packed brown sugar**
½   **cup tomato paste**
½   **cup water**
3   **garlic cloves, minced**

Combine the mustard, paprika, salt, and ¼ teaspoon of the pepper in a small bowl. Rub the seasonings onto both sides of the brisket. Cover the brisket with plastic wrap and let it stand in the refrigerator overnight.

Preheat the oven to 325 degrees F.

Heat the oil in a roasting pan just large enough to hold the brisket over medium-high heat until it's nearly smoking. Place the brisket in the pan and sear it well on both sides, about 5 minutes per side. Remove from the heat and drain off and discard the oil.

Combine the vinegar, brown sugar, tomato paste, water, garlic, and the remaining ¼ teaspoon pepper in a small saucepan over medium-high heat. Bring to a simmer and pour half of the sauce over the brisket. Set aside the remaining sauce.

Cover the roasting pan tightly with aluminum foil and bake the brisket for 4 hours, or until very tender, basting occasionally with the pan juices and adding water to the pan if necessary.

Transfer the brisket to a cutting board and slice it thickly across the grain. Return the meat to the pan, add the reserved sauce, cover the pan tightly, and reheat in the oven for 30 minutes. Serve hot.

Beef and Vegetable Stew

SERVES 6

This thick, hearty beef and fresh vegetable stew is a one-pot meal, perfect for cold winter nights. Julie Eckhert started making beef stew in college because stewing beef was inexpensive. It was also a good way to use leftover vegetables (her 1960s concept of recycling). She likes it so much that she continues to make it even though she's no longer a starving student. If you use the traditional cooking method, the aroma will fill your house and make you hungry hours in advance. When you are pressed for time, we offer a pressure-cooker shortcut.

2 **pounds beef chuck or stewing beef,**
    cut into 1-inch cubes
¼ **cup all-purpose flour**
    Salt and freshly ground pepper
3 **tablespoons canola oil**
2½–3 **cups homemade beef stock (page 59)**
2 **large onions, cut into ¼-inch-thick slices**
1 **cup chopped celery**
6 **tablespoons chopped fresh parsley**
2 **garlic cloves, minced**
½ **teaspoon dried thyme, crumbled**
6 **medium potatoes, peeled and quartered**
4 **large carrots, peeled and cut**
    into 2-inch-wide pieces
4 **medium parsnips, peeled and cut**
    into 2-inch-wide pieces
1 **cup frozen peas, thawed**

Place the beef cubes in a large bowl, add the flour and salt and pepper to taste, and toss to coat.

TRADITIONAL METHOD: Heat the oil in a large pot over medium-high heat. Add the beef cubes and brown in batches, turning, until browned on all sides, about 10 minutes. Add 2½ cups stock, the onions, celery, parsley, garlic, thyme, and salt and pepper to taste. Bring to a boil, reduce the heat to low, cover, and simmer for 2 hours. Add the potatoes, carrots, and parsnips and simmer for 1 hour more, or until the vegetables are tender. Add the peas and simmer for 5 minutes more, or until the peas are tender.

PRESSURE-COOKER METHOD: Heat the oil in a pressure cooker over medium-high heat. Add the beef cubes and brown in batches, turning, until browned on all sides, about 10 minutes. Add 3 cups stock, the onions, celery, parsley, garlic, thyme, and salt and pepper to taste. Bring to a boil, then cover and pressure-cook for 15 minutes. Add the potatoes, carrots, and parsnips and simmer, uncovered, for 1 hour, adding water if necessary. Add the peas and simmer for 5 minutes more, or until the peas are tender.

Ladle into bowls and serve.

Stuffed Pork Chops

SERVES 8

These chops are served with a quick, fresh-tasting homemade sauce instead of the usual canned-cream-soup sauce.

PORK CHOPS

8   1¼-inch-thick center-cut loin pork chops
    Salt and freshly ground pepper
1   tablespoon butter
1   tablespoon canola oil

STUFFING

1   tablespoon butter
1   tablespoon canola oil
½   cup chopped celery
4   cups cubed day-old white bread
¼   teaspoon dried sage, crumbled
    Salt and freshly ground pepper
1½ cups homemade chicken stock (page 58)
1   large egg

SAUCE

2   tablespoons butter
1   tablespoon canola oil
1   cup sliced white button mushrooms
⅔   cup evaporated skim milk
    Salt and freshly ground pepper
1   tablespoon all-purpose flour

PORK CHOPS: Preheat the oven to 350 degrees F. Season the chops with salt and pepper to taste. Heat the butter and oil in a large skillet over medium-high heat. Add the chops in batches, and sauté until browned on both sides, about 3 minutes per side. Transfer the browned chops to a 13-x-9-inch baking dish. Reserve the skillet.

STUFFING: Heat the butter and oil in the large skillet over medium heat. Add the celery and sauté until softened, about 1 minute; do not let it brown. Add the bread cubes and toss lightly. Add the sage and salt and pepper to taste. Beat the stock and the egg in a medium bowl. Add the bread mixture, toss well, and set aside.

SAUCE: Heat 1 tablespoon of the butter and the oil in the reserved skillet over medium heat. Add the mushrooms and sauté, stirring, for about 7 minutes, or until the liquid from the mushrooms evaporates. Add the evaporated milk and bring to a simmer, scraping up the browned bits from the bottom. Season with salt and pepper to taste.

Work the remaining 1 tablespoon butter and the flour into a paste in a small bowl. Whisk into the sauce over low heat a little at a time, until the sauce is thickened.

ASSEMBLY: Top each chop with about ¾ cup stuffing and pour about 1 tablespoon sauce over each chop. Bake, uncovered, for 35 minutes, or until the chops are cooked through but not dry. Serve hot.

Braised Pork Chops with Apples and Cabbage

SERVES 6

Braising meat produces a moist, flavorful dish. The onions can be omitted if they are one of your headache triggers.

6   1-inch-thick center-cut loin pork chops
     Salt and freshly ground pepper
5   tablespoons butter
2   tablespoons canola oil
12 small white onions, peeled
3   baking apples, such as Rome Beauty or Golden
        Delicious, peeled, cored, and quartered
1½ cups homemade beef stock (page 59)
1   large head green cabbage, cored and
        cut into thick wedges

Preheat the oven to 375 degrees F.

Season the chops with salt and pepper to taste. Heat 3 tablespoons of the butter and the oil in a large skillet over medium heat. Add the chops in batches and sauté until browned on both sides, about 3 minutes per side. Transfer the browned chops to a 13-x-9-inch baking dish. Add the onions to the skillet and brown on all sides, 5 to 6 minutes. With a slotted spoon, transfer the onions to the baking dish. Add the apples to the skillet and brown on both sides, about 3 minutes per side. With a slotted spoon, transfer the apples to the baking dish.

Add ¼ cup of the stock to the skillet and bring to a simmer, scraping up the browned bits from the bottom. Add the remaining 1¼ cups stock, and bring to a boil. Pour the stock mixture over the chops. Reserve the skillet. Cover the baking dish with aluminum foil and braise in the oven for 1¼ hours, or until the chops are tender.

Meanwhile, cook the cabbage in a large pot of boiling, salted water until just tender, about 10 minutes. Drain the cabbage and rinse it under cold water.

Heat the remaining 2 tablespoons butter in the reserved skillet over medium heat. Add the cabbage and sauté, stirring, for 4 minutes, or until slightly wilted. Season the cabbage with salt and pepper to taste.

When the chops are done, place the hot cabbage on a serving platter. Set the chops on top of the cabbage and arrange the apples and onions around them. Pour the juices from the baking dish over the chops and serve.

Grilled Pork Chops with Cilantro-Lime Marinade

SERVES 6

Cilantro and lime juice give this dish a
little kick of Mexican flavor.

½ cup canola oil
½ cup coarsely chopped fresh cilantro
2 teaspoons finely grated lime rind
¼ cup fresh lime juice
2 tablespoons peeled and minced fresh ginger
1 tablespoon minced garlic
1 teaspoon dry mustard
  Salt and freshly ground pepper
6 ¾-inch-thick center-cut loin pork chops

Combine the oil, cilantro, lime rind, lime juice, ginger, garlic, mustard, and salt and pepper to taste in a 13-x-9-inch baking dish.

Place the chops in the baking dish and spoon the marinade over them until the chops are mostly covered. Let stand at room temperature for 30 minutes, turning once.

Preheat an indoor or outdoor grill with a rack about 4 inches above the heat source. Remove the chops from the marinade; discard the marinade. Place the chops on the grill and cook to the desired doneness, 10 to 12 minutes per side. Serve hot.

Veal Chops with Lemon-Basil Butter

SERVES 2

This simple dish has a light, lemony flavor
that enhances the taste of the veal.

2   tablespoons butter, at room temperature
1   tablespoon finely chopped fresh basil
**   or 1 teaspoon dried, crumbled**
½   teaspoon finely grated lemon rind
1   tablespoon fresh lemon juice
2   1-inch-thick veal loin chops

Preheat the broiler.

Combine the butter, basil, lemon rind, and lemon juice in a small bowl. Hold each chop on its edge, fat side up. With a small, sharp knife, cut through the fat and halfway through the chop to create a small pocket. Stuff some of the butter mixture into each chop, then spread the remaining butter mixture on both sides of the chops.

Place the chops on a broiler pan and broil about 4 inches from the heat, turning once, for 5 to 6 minutes per side, or until browned and tender. With a fork, pierce the chop, checking often for doneness; overcooking will toughen the veal. Serve immediately.

Veal Chops with Mushroom Sauce

SERVES 4

Dry mustard spices up the mushroom sauce for these chops.
Serve over rice to soak up the sauce.

 4   1-inch-thick veal loin chops, fat trimmed
2½   tablespoons all-purpose flour
2½   tablespoons butter
10   ounces white button mushrooms, stems trimmed,
     thinly sliced
 1   cup skim milk
 1   teaspoon fresh lemon juice
 ¼   teaspoon dry mustard

Preheat the oven to 300 degrees F.

Dredge the veal chops in the flour, using as much of the flour as possible. Heat 1½ tablespoons of the butter in a large skillet over medium-low heat. Add the chops and brown for 6 to 7 minutes per side. Transfer the chops to a 9-inch square baking dish.

Heat ½ tablespoon of the butter in the skillet. Add the mushrooms and cook over medium-high heat, stirring occasionally, for 4 minutes, or until browned. With a slotted spoon, remove the mushrooms and spread over the chops, leaving behind as much of the drippings as possible. Place the baking dish in the oven to keep the veal warm while completing the sauce.

Heat the milk in a small saucepan over medium heat until hot but not boiling. Meanwhile, heat the remaining ½ tablespoon butter in the skillet over low heat, stirring to scrape up the browned bits from the bottom. Add the milk to the skillet, a little at a time, whisking constantly. Whisk in the lemon juice and mustard and simmer, whisking, for 10 minutes, or until thickened.

Pour the mushroom sauce over the chops and serve.

Roasted Veal with Gremolata

SERVES 6 TO 8

Gremolata—a mixture of chopped parsley,
garlic, and lemon rind—gives this veal dish a wonderful flavor.
The amount of lemon is well below the recommended
limits of the headache-prevention diet.

1   3-to-5-pound rolled loin of veal
1   tablespoon canola oil
    Salt and freshly ground pepper
1–1½ cups homemade chicken stock (page 58)
2   pounds small new potatoes, halved
1   pound peeled baby carrots

GREMOLATA

2   tablespoons finely chopped fresh parsley
1   garlic clove, minced
½   teaspoon finely grated lemon rind

Preheat the oven to 425 degrees F.

Rub the roast lightly with the oil and season it with salt and pepper to taste. Place the roast in a large roasting pan and pour ½ cup of the stock into the pan. Roast, uncovered, for 30 minutes.

Meanwhile, parboil the potatoes and carrots in a large saucepan of boiling water for 5 minutes. Drain.

Remove the veal from the oven, scrape up the browned bits from the pan around the meat, but leave them in the pan. Add ½ cup of the stock and the potatoes and carrots.

Reduce the oven temperature to 325 degrees F and return the roasting pan to the oven. Roast, basting with the pan juices every 15 minutes, until a meat thermometer registers 165 to 170 degrees F, 20 minutes to 1 hour. If the roast becomes dry during cooking, add another ½ cup stock.

GREMOLATA: Meanwhile, combine the parsley, garlic, and lemon rind in a small bowl.

About 10 minutes before the roast is done, remove it from the oven and press the gremolata over its surface. Baste with the pan juices and return to the oven for the last 10 minutes of cooking. Remove from the oven and let rest for 10 minutes.

Slice the veal and place on a serving platter, surround the veal with the potatoes and carrots, then pass the pan juices at the table.

Veal Landi

SERVES 8

My mom used to make this savory dish for holiday dinner parties.
It needs only rice or noodles to make a complete dinner.
Be careful not to overdo the sun-dried tomatoes.

      7 **tablespoons butter**
         Juice of 2 lemons
      2 **tablespoons canola oil**
      2 **garlic cloves, minced**
      1 **bunch broccoli, separated into small florets**
      8 **large veal cutlets (about 2 pounds total),**
            pounded to ¼ inch thick
         Salt and freshly ground pepper
         All-purpose flour
   8–12 **dry-packed sun-dried tomatoes**
      1 **cup fresh bread crumbs**
      1 **cup homemade chicken stock (page 58)**

Preheat the oven to 325 degrees F.

Melt 2 tablespoons of the butter in a 13-x-9-inch baking dish in
the oven. Remove from the oven and add ½ of the lemon juice; set
aside.

Heat 1 tablespoon of the oil and 1 tablespoon of the butter in a
large skillet over medium heat. Add the garlic and sauté until translucent, about 2 minutes. Add the broccoli and stir-fry until crisp-tender,
about 5 minutes. With a slotted spoon, transfer the garlic-broccoli
mixture to a medium bowl and set aside. Wipe out the skillet.

Season the cutlets with salt and pepper to taste and dredge them in the flour. Heat 2 tablespoons of the butter and the remaining 1 tablespoon oil in the large skillet over medium-high heat. Add the cutlets in batches and brown for 1 to 2 minutes per side. Transfer the browned cutlets to the baking dish. Reserve the skillet.

Meanwhile, blanch the sun-dried tomatoes in a small saucepan of boiling water for 10 minutes, or until softened; drain. Cut the tomatoes into ¼-inch-thick slivers. Top each cutlet with 3 or 4 tomato slivers and 3 or 4 broccoli florets. Heat the remaining 2 tablespoons butter in a small skillet over medium heat. Add the bread crumbs and sauté for 3 minutes, or until lightly browned. Sprinkle the bread crumbs over the cutlets.

Add ¼ cup of the stock to the large skillet and bring to a simmer over medium heat, scraping up the browned bits from the bottom. Add the remaining ¾ cup stock and the remaining lemon juice. Return to a simmer and cook until the sauce is reduced slightly, about 5 minutes. Pour the sauce over the veal. Cover the baking dish with aluminum foil and bake for 30 minutes, or until the veal is tender. Serve hot.

Layered Lamb Stew

SERVES 4 TO 6

Lamb stew is usually made with white wine.
Substituting chicken stock and white grape juice creates
a flavorful alternative that is safe for headache sufferers.

2 large carrots, peeled and finely chopped
2 large leeks (white parts only), washed thoroughly
    and finely chopped
3 tablespoons chopped fresh parsley
1 tablespoon minced garlic
2 pounds Yukon Gold potatoes, peeled and cut into
    ⅛-inch-thick slices
2 pounds lean lamb, cut into 1-inch cubes
    Salt and freshly ground pepper
1 cup homemade chicken stock (page 58)
½ cup white grape juice
¾ teaspoon fresh lemon juice

Preheat the oven to 350 degrees F.

Combine the carrots, leeks, parsley, and garlic in a medium bowl.

Layer one-third of the potatoes in a 3-quart baking dish. Layer half
of the carrot mixture over the potatoes, then layer half of the lamb
cubes on top of the carrot mixture. Season the lamb with salt and lots

of pepper to taste. Layer another one-third of the potatoes over the lamb, followed by the remaining carrot mixture. Layer the remaining lamb on top and season it with salt and lots of pepper to taste. Layer the remaining one-third of the potatoes on top.

Combine the stock, grape juice, and lemon juice in a small bowl. Pour the stock mixture over the stew. Cover the baking dish with aluminum foil and bake for 2½ hours. Uncover and bake for 30 minutes more, or until the top is crisp and golden. Serve hot.

Fish and Shellfish

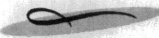

Crisp Pan-Fried Fish with Tomato and Basil

SERVES 2

The original version of this dish contained olive oil, a lot of tomatoes, and a sesame-seed coating on the fish, all of which are potential headache triggers. Our friend Julie Eckhert modified the recipe by using canola oil, reducing the amount of tomatoes, and substituting wheat germ for the sesame seeds. The result is even better than the original.

¾ pound thin whitefish fillets, such as flounder or ocean perch
  Salt
1 large egg, beaten with 1 tablespoon water
⅔ cup wheat germ or matzo meal
2 tablespoons canola oil
1 garlic clove, minced
2 small tomatoes, chopped (about 1 cup)
1 tablespoon chopped fresh basil or 1 teaspoon dried, crumbled

Season the fish with salt to taste and coat both sides with the egg mixture. Dredge the fish in the wheat germ or matzo meal, using as much of the wheat germ or matzo meal as possible. Set aside.

Heat 1 tablespoon of the oil in a large skillet over medium heat. Add the garlic and sauté, stirring, until golden, 3 to 4 minutes. Add the tomatoes and basil and sauté, stirring, until the basil wilts slightly, 1 to 2 minutes. With a slotted spoon, transfer the tomato mixture to a small bowl. Heat the remaining 1 tablespoon oil in the skillet. Add the fish and sauté for 2 to 3 minutes per side, or until it is lightly browned and flakes easily when tested with a fork. Transfer the fish to a serving platter, top with the tomato mixture, and serve.

Roast Scrod with Fresh Herbs

SERVES 2

This simple fish recipe is perfect for nights when you
don't have much time to cook, but it tastes as though you fussed
over it. The secret is the fresh herbs.

Canola oil
¾ **pound scrod, cod, or other white fish fillets**
Salt and freshly ground pepper
1½ **tablespoons melted butter**
¼ **cup mixed chopped fresh herbs (parsley, dill,**
    tarragon, and chives are a good combination;
    or oregano, basil, parsley, and garlic)
2 **tablespoons dry bread crumbs**

Preheat the oven to 450 degrees F.

Lightly oil a cookie sheet. Season the fish with salt and pepper to
taste. Place the fish on the cookie sheet and drizzle half of the butter
over the fish. Sprinkle the herbs evenly over the fish. Sprinkle the bread
crumbs evenly over the fish and drizzle with the remaining butter. Bake
the fillets for 12 to 15 minutes, or until the thickest part of each fillet
is white and flakes easily when tested with a fork. Serve immediately.

Sautéed Flounder with Cucumbers and Lime

SERVES 2

Cucumbers and fresh cilantro give this delicate fish
an exotic hint of Mexico.

¾ pound flounder or other white fish fillets
4 tablespoons fresh lime juice
½ cup all-purpose flour
     Salt and freshly ground pepper
2 tablespoons butter
2 tablespoons canola oil
2 large cucumbers, halved lengthwise, seeded,
     and thickly sliced
3 teaspoons chopped fresh cilantro
     Lime slices for garnish

Place the fish in an 8-inch square baking dish and pour 3 table-spoons of the lime juice over it. Combine the flour and salt and pepper to taste on a large plate. Dredge the fish in the flour mixture.

Heat the butter and oil in a large skillet over medium heat. Add the fish and sauté, turning once, for about 3 minutes per side, or until it is lightly browned and flakes easily when tested with a fork. Transfer the fish to a serving platter, cover with aluminum foil, and keep warm.

Add the cucumber slices to the skillet and sauté, stirring occasionally, for 6 minutes, or until lightly browned. Sprinkle the remaining 1 tablespoon lime juice and the cilantro over the fish. Arrange the cucumbers around the fish, garnish with the lime slices, and serve.

Broiled Sole with Cracker Topping

SERVES 4

Lauren Groveman, a well-known cookbook author, contributed this recipe. She says it converts even confirmed fish-haters!

7	tablespoons butter
1	cup chopped scallions
5	garlic cloves, minced
2	tablespoons fresh lemon juice
½	teaspoon crushed red pepper flakes
	Freshly ground pepper
1½	pounds sole fillets
1½	cups (1 sleeve) crushed buttery crackers, such as Ritz
	Chopped fresh parsley for garnish

Preheat the oven to 400 degrees F.

Melt 4 tablespoons of the butter in a flameproof casserole dish over medium heat. Add the scallions and garlic and sauté, stirring, until they begin to brown, 2 to 3 minutes. Let cool slightly, then stir in the lemon juice, red pepper flakes, and pepper to taste.

Dip the fillets in the scallion mixture and turn to coat them on both sides. Turn the thin ends of the fillets under to create a uniform thickness.

Melt the remaining 3 tablespoons butter in a small saucepan over low heat. Combine the melted butter and the crackers in a small bowl. Spread the cracker mixture evenly over the fish. Bake the fish for 15 minutes, then broil for 2 to 3 minutes more, or until the fish is browned and flakes easily when tested with a fork. Garnish with the parsley and serve.

Seafood Curry

SERVES 2 OR 3

The light curry sauce does not overwhelm the flavor of the seafood.
Serve with basmati, wild, or brown rice.

3   tablespoons butter
¾   pound diced lobster meat or peeled, deveined
      medium shrimp, or a mixture of both
1   cup chopped white button mushrooms
½   cup chopped onion
2   tablespoons all-purpose flour
2   cups 1% milk, heated
      Salt
1   medium apple, peeled, cored, and finely chopped
1   tablespoon curry powder

Heat 1 tablespoon of the butter in a large skillet over medium heat.
Add the lobster and/or shrimp, mushrooms, and onion and sauté, stirring, until lightly browned, about 5 minutes. Set aside.

Heat the remaining 2 tablespoons butter in a small saucepan over
low heat. Stir in the flour. Remove from the heat and gradually whisk
in 1 cup of the milk and salt to taste. Bring to a boil over medium heat.
Reduce the heat to low and simmer for 4 minutes, or until thick and
smooth, stirring constantly. Stir in the apple and curry powder. Add
the sauce to the seafood mixture and bring to a simmer over low heat.
Simmer for 20 minutes, or until heated through, stirring occasionally
and gradually adding the remaining 1 cup milk as the curry thickens.
Serve immediately.

Crab Cakes

SERVES 2 AS A MAIN DISH, 6 AS AN APPETIZER

These crab cakes are creamy inside and crunchy outside, with a bit of spiciness from the cayenne pepper. Serve as a hearty main course, or make smaller cakes and serve as an appetizer.

3 tablespoons plus 2 teaspoons butter
½ cup finely chopped celery
½ cup finely chopped scallions (white and green parts)
½ teaspoon minced garlic
1 tablespoon fresh lemon juice
2 teaspoons chopped fresh parsley
¾ teaspoon chopped fresh dill
Paprika
¼ teaspoon cayenne pepper
Salt and freshly ground pepper
2 large egg yolks
12 ounces lump crabmeat
¾ cup dry bread crumbs
3 tablespoons all-purpose flour
1⅓ cups 1% milk, heated
¼ cup canola oil
Chopped fresh parsley and lemon wedges for garnish

Heat 2 teaspoons of the butter in a large skillet over medium heat. Add the celery, scallions, and garlic and sauté, stirring, until tender, about 5 minutes. Remove from the heat.

Combine the lemon juice, parsley, dill, ½ teaspoon paprika, cayenne, and salt and pepper to taste in a small bowl. Add the lemon mixture to the skillet. Lightly beat the egg yolks in a small bowl. Add the egg yolks, crabmeat, and bread crumbs to the skillet and mix well.

Melt the remaining 3 tablespoons butter in a small saucepan over medium heat. Whisk in the flour. Add the milk a little at a time and simmer, whisking constantly, until the sauce thickens. Add salt, pepper, and paprika to taste. Stir the sauce into the crabmeat mixture. Transfer to a large bowl, cover with plastic wrap, and refrigerate for at least 30 minutes.

Form the crabmeat mixture into 6 cakes, 4 to 5 inches in diameter. Heat the oil in a large skillet over medium heat. Add the crab cakes and fry, turning once, until they are lightly browned on both sides and cooked through, about 2 minutes per side.

Sprinkle with the parsley and serve with the lemon wedges.

Garlic Shrimp

SERVES 3 OR 4

Shelling, deveining, and butterflying shrimp can be tedious. But if you pay a little extra, the fish-seller at your local market will often do it for you.

6   tablespoons (¾ stick) butter
3   garlic cloves, minced
1   pound peeled, deveined medium shrimp, butterflied
¼   cup homemade chicken stock (page 58)
1   scallion (white and green part), chopped
1   tablespoon minced fresh parsley
½   teaspoon salt
¼   teaspoon dried tarragon, crumbled
⅛   teaspoon freshly ground pepper
    Pinch nutmeg
    Pinch dried thyme, crumbled
½   cup dry bread crumbs

Preheat the oven to 400 degrees F.

Heat 4 tablespoons of the butter in a large skillet over medium heat. Add the garlic and sauté, stirring, for 1 minute, or until softened. Add half of the shrimp and sauté, stirring frequently, for about 3 minutes, or until golden brown. Transfer the shrimp to a plate and repeat with the remaining shrimp.

Return all the shrimp to the skillet and stir in the stock, scallion, parsley, salt, tarragon, pepper, nutmeg, and thyme. Transfer the shrimp mixture to a 13-x-9-inch baking dish.

Heat the 2 remaining tablespoons butter in a small skillet over low heat. Stir in the bread crumbs. Top the shrimp mixture with the bread-crumb mixture. Bake for 15 minutes, or until the top is lightly browned. Serve immediately.

Sweet and Sour Shrimp

SERVES 4

These crispy fried shrimp are served in a flavorful sweet-and-sour sauce. The bright colors of the red grapes and green pepper make the dish as appealing to the eye as it is to the palate.

2   cups water
1   cup long-grain white rice

SAUCE

1   6-ounce can tomato paste
⅓   cup sugar
¼   cup white vinegar
1   tablespoon fresh lemon juice
1   garlic clove, minced
¼   teaspoon ground ginger
1½ cups drained canned pineapple chunks,
       juice reserved
1   large green bell pepper, seeded and diced
1   cup seedless red grapes

   Canola oil
½   cup all-purpose flour
2   large eggs, lightly beaten
1½ pounds peeled, deveined large shrimp

Place the water and rice in a medium saucepan over high heat. Bring to a boil, cover, reduce the heat to low, and simmer for 20 minutes, or until the rice is tender and has absorbed all the water. Remove from the heat and set aside, covered.

SAUCE: Combine the tomato paste, sugar, vinegar, lemon juice, garlic, and ginger in a medium saucepan over medium-high heat. Bring to a boil, then add the pineapple, green pepper, and grapes. Return to a boil, reduce the heat to low, and simmer, stirring occasionally, adding small amounts of the reserved pineapple juice if the sauce gets too thick, for 15 minutes, or until slightly thickened.

Meanwhile, heat about ½ inch oil in a large skillet over medium-high heat to 350 degrees F. A cube of bread tossed in should sizzle and brown. Combine the flour, ¼ cup oil, and the eggs in a medium bowl. Dip the shrimp in the batter and deep-fry in batches until golden brown, 5 to 7 minutes. With a slotted spoon, remove the shrimp and drain on paper towels. Divide the cooked rice among 4 plates and top each portion with shrimp and a large spoonful of the sauce. Serve immediately. Pass additional sauce at the table.

Side Dishes

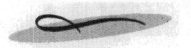

(continued on page 146)

Stir-Fried Vegetables

SERVES 4

If you're sensitive to onions, you can leave them out without compromising the flavor. Serve with rice.

2 tablespoons canola oil
4 garlic cloves, minced
2 teaspoons peeled and grated fresh ginger
1 medium onion, thinly sliced
1 teaspoon sugar
5 ounces white button mushrooms, stems trimmed, thinly sliced
1 medium zucchini, trimmed and cut into ¼-inch-thick slices
1 cup bite-size broccoli florets
1 teaspoon salt
1 medium tomato, chopped

Heat the oil in a large skillet or wok over medium heat. Add the garlic and ginger and sauté, stirring, until the garlic is translucent, about 3 minutes. Add the onion and sugar and sauté, stirring frequently, until the onion is caramelized, 2 to 3 minutes. Be careful not to let it burn. Increase the heat to medium-high, add the mushrooms, and stir-fry until they give up their juices, 4 to 5 minutes.

Add the zucchini, broccoli, and salt and stir-fry until they are crisp-tender, about 4 minutes more. Add the tomato and stir-fry until heated through, about 1 minute. Serve hot.

Roasted Asparagus and Mushrooms with Herbs

SERVES 4

I first served this easy-to-make dish at a dinner party. I knew it was a success when three of my guests asked for the recipe.

1	pound asparagus, ends snapped off
8–10	ounces white button mushrooms, stems trimmed
2	medium tomatoes, each cored and cut into 8 wedges
2	teaspoons canola oil
¼	teaspoon dried rosemary, crumbled
¼	teaspoon dried thyme, crumbled
	Freshly ground pepper

Preheat the oven to 500 degrees F.

Combine the asparagus, mushrooms, tomatoes, oil, rosemary, thyme, and pepper to taste in a large bowl. Toss well.

Arrange the vegetables in a single layer on a cookie sheet. Bake, stirring occasionally, for 10 minutes, or until the asparagus is crisp-tender. Serve.

Candied Carrots

SERVES 6

These candied carrots are a more interesting alternative to the ubiquitous candied yams served at most Thanksgiving dinners.

3 cups peeled and grated carrots
¼ cup dark brown sugar
4 tablespoons (½ stick) butter

Combine the carrots, brown sugar, and butter in a large skillet over medium heat. When the butter begins to melt, stir, cover, reduce the heat to low, and cook, stirring occasionally, until the carrots are very tender and lightly glazed, about 15 minutes. Serve hot.

Creamed Beets with Dill

SERVES 4

The original version of this dish was made with sour cream. Since sour cream is not allowed on the headache-prevention diet, I substituted cream cheese and low-fat milk. The result is excellent.

1½ **pounds fresh beets, peeled and cut
    into ½-inch cubes**
¼ **cup cream cheese**
2 **tablespoons butter**
1 **cup 1% milk
    Salt and freshly ground pepper**
2 **tablespoons chopped fresh dill or 2 teaspoons
    dried, crumbled**

Place the beets in a large saucepan over high heat and add water to cover. Bring to a boil, reduce the heat to medium, and simmer until tender, 10 to 20 minutes. Drain and set aside.

Heat the cream cheese and butter in a large skillet over medium heat until melted. Whisk in the milk and cook, whisking, for about 3 minutes, or until the sauce is smooth. Add the beets, season with salt and pepper to taste, and cook, stirring, until the beets are heated through, about 5 minutes. Stir in the dill and serve.

Jewish-Style Baby Artichokes

SERVES 4 TO 6

This recipe, handed down from David's grandmother,
is elegant in its simplicity.

12 2-inch-long baby artichokes
Juice of 2 lemons
Salt and freshly ground pepper
Canola oil

Cut the stems off the artichokes and cut ½ inch off the tips.

Place each artichoke upside down on a work surface and press down so that the leaves spread out. Rinse the artichokes thoroughly with cold water. Season the artichokes with the lemon juice and salt and pepper to taste.

Place 1 inch of oil in a large skillet over medium-low heat. Place the artichokes in the skillet upside down with the leaves spread out and sauté, turning once, for 8 minutes, or until browned and crisp.

Serve warm.

French-Fried Eggplant

SERVES 3 OR 4

Here's a great way to get children to eat eggplant:
Disguise it as french fries. These crispy strips disappear as
quickly as you can say, "Pass the salt!"

1   **large eggplant, peeled**
    1% milk
    All-purpose flour
    Canola oil
    Salt

Slice the eggplant into 1-inch-thick rounds, then cut the rounds
into long french-fry strips. Place the eggplant strips in a medium bowl,
add milk to cover, and let stand for 30 minutes. Put a generous amount
of flour in a zipper-lock plastic bag, add the eggplant strips, and shake
until the strips are coated with the flour. Transfer the strips to a large
colander and shake off the excess flour over the sink.

Heat ½ inch of oil in a large skillet over medium-high heat to 350
degrees F. A cube of bread tossed in will sizzle and brown. Add the eggplant strips and fry, turning, until golden brown on all sides, about 10
minutes. Drain on paper towels. Season with salt to taste and serve.

Eggplant Italiano

SERVES 4

This is a great Italian-style dish with only a small—and
headache-safe—amount of tomato per serving.

1 **large egg**
1 **cup fresh bread crumbs (from about 4 slices bread)**
1 **large eggplant, cut into ½-inch-thick rounds**
  Canola oil
1–2 **tablespoons butter**
1 **medium tomato, chopped**
¼ **cup homemade vegetable stock (page 60)**
½ **teaspoon minced fresh oregano or ¼ teaspoon**
  dried, crumbled
½ **teaspoon minced fresh basil or ¼ teaspoon dried,**
  crumbled
  Salt and freshly ground pepper

Beat the egg in a wide, shallow bowl and place the bread crumbs
on a large plate. Dip the eggplant rounds in the egg, then dredge in the
bread crumbs.

Heat 1 tablespoon oil and 1 tablespoon butter in a large skillet over
medium heat. Add the eggplant and sauté in batches, adding more oil
and butter as needed, turning once, until golden brown and tender,
about 10 minutes. Drain on paper towels. Transfer the eggplant to a
warm serving platter. Cover with aluminum foil and keep warm.

Heat 1 tablespoon oil in the large skillet over medium heat. Add
the tomato, stock, oregano, basil, and salt and pepper to taste and sauté
until slightly thickened, 8 to 10 minutes. Pour over the eggplant and
serve warm.

Stuffed Eggplant

SERVES 4

This is a terrific vegetarian side dish or main course.
The eggplants make natural baking "dishes" that
hold the creamy vegetable filling.

2	medium eggplants, halved lengthwise
4	tablespoons (½ stick) butter
2	tablespoons canola oil
2	cups fresh bread crumbs (from about 8 slices bread)
½	cup finely chopped onion
2	garlic cloves, minced
1½	cups finely chopped white button mushrooms
1½	cups finely chopped zucchini
¼	cup chopped fresh parsley
1	tablespoon chopped fresh basil
1	teaspoon chopped fresh oregano or ½ teaspoon dried, crumbled
	Salt and freshly ground pepper
½	cup part-skim ricotta cheese

Preheat the oven to 350 degrees F.

Scoop out the flesh from the insides of the eggplants and cut it into ½-inch cubes. (You should have 1½ cups.) Set aside the eggplant skins and flesh.

Heat 3 tablespoons of the butter and 1 tablespoon of the oil in a large skillet over medium heat. Add the bread crumbs and sauté, stirring occasionally, until lightly browned, about 5 minutes. Transfer the bread crumbs to a small bowl and set aside. Wipe out the skillet.

Heat the remaining 1 tablespoon oil and the remaining 1 table-spoon butter in the large skillet over medium heat. Add the onion and garlic and sauté, stirring occasionally, until the onion is translucent, about 5 minutes. Add the mushrooms and sauté, stirring, for 3 minutes more. Add the zucchini and the eggplant cubes and sauté, stirring, until everything is tender, about 10 minutes. Stir in the parsley, basil, oregano, and salt and pepper to taste.

Add the bread crumbs to the vegetable mixture, reduce the heat to low, and cook for 2 minutes, or until heated through. Remove from the heat and stir in the ricotta cheese. Spoon the vegetable mixture into the eggplant skins. Place the stuffed eggplants on a cookie sheet. Bake for 25 minutes, or until the tops are browned. Serve immediately.

Stuffed Green Peppers

SERVES 4

As long as you don't use freshly baked bread,
this classic dish is perfect for the headache sufferer.

4 **medium green bell peppers, halved lengthwise, stemmed, and seeded**
8 **slices whole wheat bread, cut into ¼-inch cubes**
6 **tablespoons (¾ stick) butter**
4 **garlic cloves, minced**
3 **tablespoons chopped fresh parsley**
2 **tablespoons chopped fresh oregano**
   Salt and freshly ground pepper

Preheat the oven to 400 degrees F.

Place the green pepper halves skin side down in a single layer in a 13-x-9-inch baking dish and add ½ inch of water to the dish.

Place the bread cubes in a medium bowl. Heat the butter in a small skillet over medium heat. Add the garlic and sauté until browned, about 3 minutes. Stir in the parsley, oregano, and salt and pepper to taste. Add the butter mixture to the bread cubes and toss well.

Stuff the pepper halves with the bread mixture. Cover the baking dish with aluminum foil and bake for 15 minutes. Uncover and bake for about 15 minutes more, or until the peppers are soft and the stuffing is lightly browned. Serve hot.

Sautéed Turnips with Mustard

SERVES 4 TO 6

This tangy side dish is easy to prepare and is a pleasant
alternative to more standard recipes.

1½ **pounds small turnips, peeled and cut
into 1-inch chunks
Salt**
2 **tablespoons butter**
1 **tablespoon dry mustard, dissolved in
1 tablespoon water**
2 **tablespoons chopped fresh parsley**

Place the turnips and salt to taste in a large saucepan over high
heat, add water to cover, and bring to a boil. Reduce the heat to medium and simmer until tender, 12 to 15 minutes. Drain well.

Heat the butter in a large skillet over medium heat. Stir in the mustard mixture. Add the turnips and salt to taste and cook, stirring, until
the turnips are heated through and thoroughly coated with the mustard mixture, about 5 minutes. Stir in the parsley and serve hot.

Baked Acorn Squash

SERVES 4

With its sturdy texture and sweet flavor, this fresh winter squash
is far more interesting than the frozen kind.

1   **large acorn squash, halved crosswise and seeded**
4   **teaspoons light brown sugar**
4   **teaspoons butter**
    Salt

Preheat the oven to 425 degrees F.

Fill the hollow in each squash half with 2 teaspoons of the brown
sugar, 2 teaspoons of the butter, and salt to taste. Place the squash in a
baking dish and add ½ inch water to the dish. Cover with aluminum
foil and bake for 45 minutes. Uncover and bake for 20 minutes more,
or until the squash can be pierced easily with a fork. Cut each squash
half in half again. Baste with the pan juices and serve warm.

Broccoli Pancakes

MAKES 20 PANCAKES; SERVES 4 OR 5

My mother created this variation on classic potato latkes
(page 36). Our kids love it—it's the only way we
can get them to eat broccoli.

1 **bunch broccoli (about 1¼ pounds), separated
   into florets and stems**
3 **large eggs**
½ **cup all-purpose flour**
1 **teaspoon salt**
  Freshly ground pepper
  Canola oil

Preheat the oven to 250 degrees F.

Puree 1 cup of the broccoli florets in a food processor. Transfer to
a small bowl and set aside. Shred enough of the broccoli stems in the
food processor, using the shredding blade, to equal 1 cup.

Beat the eggs in a medium bowl. Whisk in the flour, salt, and pepper to taste. Whisk in the pureed and shredded broccoli.

Heat ½ inch of oil in a large skillet over medium-high heat to 350
degrees F. A cube of bread tossed in should sizzle and brown. Drop
heaping tablespoons of the broccoli mixture into the skillet; do not
crowd. Fry in batches, turning once, until browned, about 5 minutes
per side. Transfer the pancakes to paper towels to drain. Place the pancakes on a cookie sheet in the oven while you cook the remaining pancakes. Serve hot.

Tsimmis

SERVES 8

This recipe was handed down from David's grandmother.
It's traditionally served at the beginning of the Jewish New Year,
because its sweetness is supposed to guarantee a full and
sweet year ahead. But there's no reason to serve it
just once a year. Be careful not to overindulge, or you'll risk
exceeding the ½-cup-per-day limit on pineapple.

2   **16-ounce cans yams, drained**
1   **16-ounce can whole tiny carrots, drained**
1   **16-ounce can pineapple chunks, drained,**
     ½ cup juice reserved
2   **small apples, peeled, cored, and cut into**
     ¼-inch-thick slices
½   **cup light brown sugar**
2   **tablespoons butter**
½   **teaspoon ground cinnamon**
¼   **teaspoon salt**
⅛   **teaspoon ground ginger**

Preheat the oven to 350 degrees F.

Layer half of the yams in a 9-inch square baking dish. Top with half of the carrots, half of the pineapple, and half of the apples.

Using a fork, mash the brown sugar, butter, cinnamon, salt, and ginger in a small bowl.

Sprinkle half of the brown-sugar mixture on top of the apples, then top with the remaining yams, the remaining carrots, the remaining pineapple, and the remaining apples. Sprinkle the remaining brown-sugar mixture on top.

Pour the reserved pineapple juice into the baking dish. Cover and bake for 1 hour. Uncover and bake until the top is browned, about 10 minutes. Serve warm.

Jack-Be-Little Pumpkin Timbales

SERVES 8

This dish is especially appropriate for a Halloween or Thanksgiving dinner. If you can't find the miniature Jack-Be-Little pumpkins, you can use custard cups instead.

- 8 Jack-Be-Little pumpkins (make sure they're edible, not ornamental)
- 2 large butternut squashes, peeled and cut into 4-inch chunks
- 2 medium sweet potatoes
- 1½ cups evaporated skim milk
- 4 large eggs
- 1 teaspoon salt
- ½ teaspoon paprika
- 4 tablespoons (½ stick) butter
- 2 tablespoons light brown sugar

Preheat the oven to 350 degrees F.

Cut 1-inch circles out of the tops of the pumpkins and scoop out and discard the seeds and strings. Place the pumpkins and their tops, stem side up, in a large roasting pan. Cover with aluminum foil and bake for 20 minutes, or until the pumpkins can be easily pierced with a fork. Set the pumpkins aside in the roasting pan.

Place the squash and sweet potatoes in a 13-x-9-inch baking dish and bake for 1 hour, or until tender when pierced with a fork. Peel the sweet potatoes when they are cool to the touch, then cut the potatoes and squash into ½-inch cubes. (You should have about 2½ cups squash and 1 cup sweet potatoes.) Set aside the sweet potatoes and 1 cup of the squash. Reduce the oven temperature to 325 degrees F.

Puree 1½ cups of the squash in a food processor. Add the evaporated milk, eggs, ¾ teaspoon of the salt, and the paprika and process to combine. Pour the squash mixture into the pumpkins until they are three-fourths full. Bake for 40 to 50 minutes, or until a knife inserted into the filling comes out clean.

Meanwhile, place the remaining 1 cup squash, the sweet potatoes, butter, brown sugar, and the remaining ¼ teaspoon salt in a medium skillet over medium heat. Sauté for 3 to 4 minutes, stirring, until the butter and sugar are melted and everything is heated through.

Place the timbale-filled pumpkins on a serving platter. Top each pumpkin with about ¼ cup of the sweet-potato mixture. Set the pumpkin tops on the pumpkins and serve hot.

Corn Pudding

SERVES 4

This "pudding" is a side dish, not a dessert.
The recipe comes from Priscilla Alden van Cott, who says
it's been served at every Thanksgiving in her family since
just after the Revolutionary War.

5½ **tablespoons butter, at room temperature**
2 **cups fresh corn kernels or 10 ounces frozen
       corn, thawed**
¾ **cup 1% milk**
2 **large eggs**
1½ **tablespoons sugar**
1 **tablespoon all-purpose flour**
¾ **teaspoon salt**

Preheat the oven to 350 degrees F.

Butter a 13-x-9-inch baking dish with ½ tablespoon of the butter. Puree the corn, milk, eggs, 4 tablespoons of the butter, sugar, flour, and salt in a food processor for 10 seconds. It will be chunky. Pour the corn mixture into the baking dish and dot it with the remaining 1 tablespoon butter. Bake for 45 minutes, or until a knife inserted in the center comes out clean. Serve immediately.

Caesar Salad

SERVES 8

Traditional Caesar salad is forbidden on the headache-prevention diet because of the anchovies and aged cheese. But this version tastes exactly like the real thing. Be sure to use a very fresh egg. You can also prepare this salad without the raw egg yolk.

¾ **cup canola oil**
3 **dry-packed sun-dried tomatoes, minced**
1 **garlic clove, minced, plus 1 whole garlic clove**
1 **teaspoon salt**
¼ **teaspoon dry mustard**
   Freshly ground pepper
5 **tablespoons fresh lemon juice**
1 **large egg yolk**
4 **slices white bread, cut into ½-inch cubes**
1 **head romaine lettuce, washed and torn into**
   bite-size pieces

Combine ½ cup of the oil, the sun-dried tomatoes, and the minced garlic in a small bowl and let stand for 20 minutes. Add the salt, mustard, and a generous grinding of pepper to taste and mash into a paste. Beat the lemon juice and egg yolk in a small bowl. Whisk the lemon-juice mixture into the oil mixture.

Heat the remaining ¼ cup oil in a medium skillet over medium heat. Add the garlic clove and sauté for 3 minutes, or until browned; remove and discard the garlic. Add the bread cubes to the skillet and sauté, stirring, until brown on all sides, about 5 minutes. With a slotted spoon, transfer the croutons to paper towels to drain.

Place the lettuce in a large salad bowl and toss with the dressing. Add the croutons, toss again, and serve immediately.

Beet and Mango Salad with Curried Mango Dressing

SERVES 8

This distinctive spicy-sweet salad draws "oohs" and "aahs" every time it's served. The purple beets on the dark green lettuce are a beautiful color combination. Serve with roast chicken or braised lamb chops.

CURRIED MANGO DRESSING

1½ ripe mangoes, peeled, pitted, and finely chopped
⅓ cup white vinegar
1½ tablespoons pure maple syrup
1½ teaspoons dry mustard, dissolved in 1½ teaspoons
     water
1 teaspoon curry powder
    Salt
½ cup canola oil

SALAD

6 medium beets, tops removed
⅔ cup diced red onion
1 head romaine lettuce
1½ ripe mangoes, peeled, pitted, and cut
     into long strips

DRESSING: Combine the mango, vinegar, maple syrup, mustard mixture, curry powder, and salt to taste in a food processor and process until smooth. Add the oil and process until emulsified.

SALAD: Place the beets in a large plastic bag; do not seal. Microwave on high for 18 minutes, turning the bag twice, until the beets can be easily pierced with a knife. (Or, to cook the beets on the stovetop, place them in a medium saucepan, add water to cover, and boil for 30 to 45 minutes, or until tender. Drain.) Let the beets cool slightly, then rinse them with cold water. Peel the beets and cut them into ¾-inch cubes.

Toss the beets with ¼ cup of the dressing in a medium bowl. Let stand at room temperature for 30 minutes, then stir in the onion.

Place 4 lettuce leaves on each of 8 plates. Spoon the beets onto the lettuce and arrange the mango strips over and around the beets. Pour more dressing on top. Serve immediately, passing the remaining dressing at the table.

Lemon - Tarragon Salad Dressing

MAKES 1 CUP

Headache-safe salads are hard to come by, owing to the difficulty of finding a dressing that does not contain forbidden aged cheeses, vinegars, or prepared mustards. This dressing uses just a little lemon juice and is excellent over baby spinach or arugula.

- ¾ cup canola oil
- ¼ cup fresh lemon juice
- 2 garlic cloves, minced
- 2 teaspoons dried tarragon, crumbled
- 1½ teaspoons dry mustard
- 1 teaspoon salt
- ¼ teaspoon freshly ground pepper

Whisk together all the ingredients in a small bowl. Use immediately, or cover and refrigerate for up to 10 days.

Mashed Sweet Potatoes

SERVES 6 TO 8

The latest research suggests that sweet potatoes are
more nutritious than white potatoes. This dish isn't too sweet,
and it's quick enough to make on weeknights.

5 **medium sweet potatoes**
⅓ **cup skim milk**
4 **tablespoons (½ stick) butter**
1 **tablespoon light brown sugar**
½ **teaspoon salt**
   Ground cinnamon

Preheat the oven to 375 degrees F.

Cook the sweet potatoes in a large pot of boiling water until tender when pierced with a knife, 30 to 45 minutes. Drain. Peel the sweet potatoes as soon as they are cool enough to handle. Slice the potatoes and place them in a large bowl. Add the milk, 3 tablespoons of the butter, the brown sugar, salt, and ¼ teaspoon cinnamon. Beat with an electric mixer until smooth. Transfer to a 13-x-9-inch baking dish and dot with the remaining 1 tablespoon butter. Sprinkle with cinnamon to taste. Bake for 10 minutes, or until heated through and the top is browned. Serve hot.

Mashed Potatoes with Parsnip and Garlic

SERVES 4 TO 6

A parsnip gives these mashed potatoes a special flavor.

- 4 large russet potatoes, peeled and cut into ½-inch cubes
- 1 medium parsnip, peeled and cut into ½-inch cubes
- 4 garlic cloves, unpeeled
- 1 teaspoon canola oil
- ½ cup skim milk
- 2 tablespoons butter

Preheat the oven to 350 degrees F.

Cook the potatoes and parsnip in a large pot of boiling water until they are soft, about 15 minutes. Drain and transfer to a large bowl.

Meanwhile, cut off and discard 1 end from each garlic clove and place the garlic in a small baking dish. Drizzle with the oil and bake for 30 minutes, or until soft. Let cool for 1 minute, then squeeze the garlic cloves out of the skins. Gently crush the cloves with the flat side of a knife.

Add the garlic, milk, and butter to the potatoes and parsnip and beat with an electric mixer until smooth. Serve immediately.

Rosemary Scalloped Potatoes

SERVES 4

These scalloped potatoes are creamy, with a rich brown crust.
This dish is simple to prepare, especially if you
slice the potatoes with a food processor.

4   cups thinly sliced peeled potatoes (about
       5 medium potatoes)
     Salt
¼   cup chopped scallions
1½ teaspoons chopped fresh rosemary or ½ teaspoon
       dried, crumbled
1   tablespoon butter
1½ cups 1% milk, heated
½   cup wheat germ
¼   teaspoon paprika

Preheat the oven to 350 degrees F.

Place the potato slices in a 13-x-9-inch baking dish and season
with salt to taste. Add the scallions and rosemary and mix well. Dot
with the butter and pour the milk over the top. Sprinkle the wheat
germ and paprika on top. Bake for 1¼ hours, or until the top is
browned. Serve hot.

Mushroom-Stuffed Baked Potatoes

SERVES 6

This side dish can also be a light meal.
One-percent milk gives creaminess without cream.

6   large russet potatoes
2   tablespoons butter
1   tablespoon canola oil
1   pound white button mushrooms, finely chopped
1   medium onion, chopped
    Pinch of nutmeg
    Salt and freshly ground pepper
1   large egg yolk, lightly beaten
1   tablespoon 1% milk

Preheat the oven to 450 degrees F.

Bake the potatoes for 1 hour, or until they can be pierced easily with a fork. Set aside.

Heat 1 tablespoon of the butter and the oil in a large skillet over low heat. Add the mushrooms and onion and sauté, stirring occasionally, for 10 minutes, or until browned. Season with the nutmeg and salt and pepper to taste. Stir in the egg yolk and remove from the heat.

Preheat the broiler.

Halve the potatoes lengthwise and scoop out half of the flesh. Place the flesh in a medium bowl and stir in the mushroom mixture and the milk. Stuff the potatoes with the potato-mushroom mixture and place a small piece of the remaining 1 tablespoon butter on top of each. Broil for 10 minutes, or until the tops are browned. Serve immediately.

Mushroom Rice Pilaf

SERVES 4

Rice pilaf sometimes contains almonds, which can be headache triggers. The mushrooms in this recipe add plenty of flavor.

- 1½ **tablespoons butter**
- 8 **ounces white button mushrooms, chopped**
- 1 **cup long-grain white rice**
- 2½ **cups homemade chicken stock (page 58), heated**

Heat the butter in a large skillet over medium heat. Add the mushrooms and sauté, stirring occasionally, until softened, 7 to 8 minutes. Add the rice and sauté, stirring, until it is golden, 5 to 7 minutes. Add the stock and bring to a boil. Reduce the heat to low, cover, and simmer until all the stock is absorbed, 15 to 20 minutes. Fluff with a fork and serve.

Mexican Rice

SERVES 6 TO 8

Because they contain aged cheese or a lot of tomato, many Mexican dishes are forbidden to headache sufferers. This great side dish with a Latin flavor limits the tomato to a small amount per serving. Serve with Mexican Chicken (page 98).

4 **cups homemade chicken stock (page 58)**
1½ **cups brown basmati rice**
1 **tablespoon chili powder**
½ **teaspoon ground cumin**
1 **tablespoon canola oil**
1 **cup fresh corn kernels or 1 cup frozen, thawed**
1 **cup diced green bell pepper**
½ **cup diced red bell pepper**
½ **cup diced yellow bell pepper**
1 **cup diced tomato**
2 **tablespoons chopped fresh cilantro**
2 **teaspoons fresh lime juice**

Place the stock in a large saucepan over high heat and bring to a boil. Add the rice, chili powder, and cumin and return to a boil. Reduce the heat to low, cover, and simmer until the rice is tender and the stock is absorbed, about 15 minutes.

Meanwhile, heat the oil in a large skillet over medium heat. Add the corn and bell peppers and sauté, stirring, for 4 minutes, or until crisp-tender. Add the tomato and sauté for 2 minutes more, or until heated through. Stir the vegetable mixture, cilantro, and lime juice into the rice mixture and serve.

Rice with Asparagus and Sun-Dried Tomatoes

SERVES 8

This colorful dish is an excellent foil for some of the spicier dishes in this book, such as Garlic Shrimp (page 140) or Steak au Poivre (page 111).

- 1 bunch asparagus, ends snapped off, cut diagonally into thirds
- 4 cups water
- 2 tablespoons finely chopped dry-packed sun-dried tomatoes
- 1 tablespoon butter
- 2¼ teaspoons salt
- 2 cups long-grain white rice
- 1 teaspoon canola oil
- ¼ teaspoon freshly ground pepper

Steam the asparagus in a steamer basket in a large saucepan over 1 inch of boiling water for 3 to 4 minutes, or until crisp-tender. Transfer the asparagus to an icewater bath. Drain and transfer to a medium bowl and set aside.

Meanwhile, place the 4 cups of water, sun-dried tomatoes, butter, and 1 teaspoon of the salt in a medium saucepan over high heat and bring to a boil. Add the rice and return to a boil. Reduce the heat to low, cover, and simmer for 15 to 20 minutes, or until tender and all the water is absorbed.

Toss the asparagus with 1 teaspoon of the salt and the oil. Add the asparagus to the rice mixture and toss well. Season with the remaining ¼ teaspoon salt and the pepper. Serve hot.

Desserts

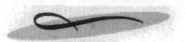

New Orleans–Style Bread Pudding

SERVES 10 TO 12

This dessert is light and fluffy, yet still moist. The thinly sliced apples melt into the pudding, giving it a subtle sweetness.

- 1 1-pound loaf day-old French bread
- 4 cups skim milk
   About 10 tablespoons (1¼ sticks) unsalted butter
- 4 large eggs
- 1½ cups sugar
- 4 teaspoons vanilla extract
- 2 large Granny Smith apples, peeled, cored, and cut into paper-thin slices
- 1 cup confectioners' sugar

Crumble the bread into a large bowl. Pour the milk over it and let stand for 1 hour.

Preheat the oven to 325 degrees F, with a rack in the middle. Butter a 13-x-9-inch baking dish, using 1 to 2 tablespoons of the butter.

Beat together 3 of the eggs, the sugar, and 2 teaspoons of the vanilla in a small bowl. Add to the bread mixture and stir well.

Place a layer of one-fourth of the bread mixture in the baking dish. Top with one-third of the apples. Add another layer of one-fourth of the bread mixture, and top with one-third of the apples. Continue, making another layer of bread and apples, and ending with a final layer of bread.

Bake the pudding for 60 to 70 minutes, or until browned and set. Let the pudding cool to room temperature.

Preheat the broiler.

Combine the remaining 8 to 9 tablespoons butter and the confectioners' sugar in a double boiler over simmering water and cook, stirring, until the sugar is dissolved and the mixture is very hot. Remove from the heat.

Whisk together the remaining 1 egg and the remaining 2 teaspoons vanilla in a small bowl, then whisk the egg mixture into the sugar mixture. Whisk constantly until the sauce has cooled to room temperature.

Cut the pudding into 10 to 12 servings and place in a broilerproof pan. Spoon the sauce over the pudding and broil until bubbly, about 5 minutes. Serve immediately.

Frozen Lemon Torte

SERVES 8

This frozen dessert has a texture somewhere between cheesecake and ice cream. The zesty lemon flavor makes a perfect ending to a hearty meal. The torte can be prepared in advance.

CRUST

16 ounces (about 1½ boxes) vanilla wafers
6 tablespoons unsalted butter, melted

FILLING

6 large eggs, 3 separated
1¼ cups plus 3 tablespoons sugar
1 teaspoon finely grated lemon rind
½ cup fresh lemon juice

TOPPING

3 large egg whites
1 tablespoon sugar

CRUST: Chop the vanilla wafers into fine crumbs in a food processor. Transfer the crumbs to a small bowl and stir in the butter. Press the wafer mixture into an 8-inch springform pan, covering the bottom and sides and pressing down firmly. Set aside.

FILLING: In a double boiler over simmering water, combine the 3 eggs, 3 egg yolks, 1¼ cups of the sugar, the lemon rind, and lemon juice. Cook, stirring constantly, until thickened, about 10 minutes. Remove from the heat and let cool to room temperature, then cover tightly with plastic wrap.

Beat the 3 egg whites in a medium bowl until foamy. Add the

remaining 3 tablespoons sugar and beat until stiff. Fold the egg-white mixture into the lemon mixture. Pour the filling into the crust. Freeze for at least 5 hours or overnight.

TOPPING: Preheat the broiler. Beat the egg whites in a medium bowl until foamy. Add the sugar and beat until stiff. Pour over the filling. Broil until the top is golden—this will take just 1 to 3 minutes, so watch carefully. Return the torte to the freezer to set, about 6 hours. Remove the torte from the freezer to soften about 15 minutes before serving. Cut the torte into wedges and serve.

Apple-Cranberry Crisp

SERVES 8

Cranberries give this apple crisp a tart
contrast to the standard version.

1   cup sugar
1   cup water
2   cups fresh cranberries, picked over
6½ tablespoons unsalted butter, at room temperature
8   Granny Smith apples, peeled, cored, and each cut
    into 8–10 slices
1   cup light brown sugar
¼   teaspoon ground cinnamon
¾   cup all-purpose flour
¼   teaspoon salt

Preheat the oven to 375 degrees F.

Place the sugar and water in a medium saucepan over medium-
high heat and bring to a boil, stirring. Add the cranberries, reduce the
heat to low, and simmer for about 5 minutes, or until the cranberries
are tender and pop. Drain.

Butter a 9-inch pie pan or an 8-inch square baking dish, using ½
tablespoon of the butter. Toss together the apples and cranberries in the
prepared pan or dish. Combine ½ cup of the brown sugar and the cinnamon in a small bowl and sprinkle over the fruit.

Place the remaining ½ cup of brown sugar, the flour, and salt in a
food processor and pulse to mix. Add the remaining 6 tablespoons butter and pulse until the mixture forms small crumbs; do not overprocess,
or it will clump together.

Sprinkle the crumb mixture over the apples and cranberries. Bake
for 45 minutes, or until the apples are tender and the top is browned.
Serve warm.

Crater Cookies

MAKES 2 DOZEN

Our friend Julie Luchs volunteered her grandmother's
recipe for "the best butter cookies you've ever tasted."
After trying them, I had to agree.

16	tablespoons (2 sticks) unsalted butter, at room temperature
1	cup sugar
2	large egg yolks
2½	cups sifted flour
1	teaspoon vanilla extract
¼	teaspoon salt
	About ¼ cup jam or jelly

Preheat the oven to 350 degrees F.

Beat the butter with an electric mixer in a large bowl until soft, about 5 minutes. Add the sugar and beat until fluffy. Beat in the egg yolks, one at a time. Add the flour, vanilla, and salt and stir until well blended.

Shape the dough into 1-inch balls, and place them 2 inches apart on 2 ungreased cookie sheets. With your thumb, make an indentation in each dough ball and place about ½ teaspoon jam or jelly in the "crater." Bake for 12 to 15 minutes, or until golden brown. Cool the cookies on a rack. Store for up to 2 weeks in an airtight container.

Lemon Meringue Cookies

MAKES ABOUT 2½ DOZEN

Our friends always ask me to bring these
cookies to their parties. They didn't know how easy
these cookies are to make . . . until now.

5   **egg whites, at room temperature**
1   **teaspoon vanilla extract**
1½ **cups superfine sugar**
1   **13-ounce jar lemon curd (about 1¼ cups)**

Preheat the oven to 450 degrees F.

Beat the egg whites and vanilla with an electric mixer in a large
bowl until soft peaks form. Gradually add the sugar and beat until stiff
peaks form.

Line a cookie sheet with aluminum foil and draw 2-inch circles on
the foil. Cover the circles with the meringue mixture, spreading about
½-inch deep. Using a pastry bag with a ¼-inch tip, pipe a border
around the edge of the circles to build up the sides of the cookies.

Turn off the oven and place the meringues in the oven for at least
5 hours, or until hardened. Fill each meringue with about 2 teaspoons
lemon curd. Store the cookies in an airtight container for up to 1 week.

Palmiers with Vanilla Glaze

MAKES 4 TO 5 DOZEN

These impressive cookies are beautiful and they won't
give you a headache.

3   **tablespoons unsalted butter**
1   **17.3-ounce package frozen puff-pastry dough**
    Sugar
2½ **tablespoons 1% milk**
½   **teaspoon vanilla extract**
1½ **cups confectioners' sugar, sifted**
    Pinch salt

Preheat the oven to 375 degrees F. Butter 4 cookie sheets, using 2
tablespoons of the butter.

Roll out each sheet of pastry on a sugared surface into an 11-x-10-
inch rectangle, about ⅛ inch thick. Fold the longer sides of each rectangle into the center, leaving about ¼ inch uncovered down the center of the rectangles in the folded edges to meet in the center, forming
an 11-inch-long log. Cut each log crosswise into wide slices. Sprinkle
the rectangles with sugar and place about 2 inches apart on the cookie
sheets.

Bake for 5 minutes, then turn the cookies and bake for 3 to 5 minutes more, or until the edges begin to turn golden brown. Immediately
transfer the cookies to racks to cool.

Melt the remaining 1 tablespoon butter in a small saucepan over
low heat, then remove from the heat and stir in the milk and vanilla.
Add the confectioners' sugar and salt and stir until smooth.

When the cookies are cool, dip one end of each cookie into the
glaze. Let the cookies stand on wax paper until the glaze is firm. Store
for up to 1 week in an airtight container.

Moist Orange Pound Cake

SERVES 12 TO 16

Orange enhances the flavor of this pound cake.
Despite the "citrusy" flavor, this dessert conforms to the
recommended limits for citrus fruits.

CAKE

1¼   cups (2½ sticks) plus 1 tablespoon unsalted butter,
       at room temperature
3   cups plus 2 tablespoons all-purpose flour, sifted
2¾   cups sugar
5   large eggs
1   teaspoon orange extract
1   teaspoon vanilla extract
1   teaspoon baking powder
¼   teaspoon salt
¼   cup evaporated skim milk
¾   cup orange juice
1½   tablespoons finely grated orange rind

CITRUS SOAK

¾   cup confectioners' sugar
¾   cup orange juice
½   teaspoon fresh lemon juice

Preheat the oven to 350 degrees F. Butter and flour a 12-cup bundt pan, using 1 tablespoon of the butter and 2 tablespoons of the flour.

C A K E : Beat the remaining 1¼ cups butter, the sugar, eggs, orange extract, and vanilla with an electric mixer on low speed in a large bowl for 30 seconds, scraping the sides of the bowl as needed. Beat on high for 5 minutes, or until slightly fluffy, scraping down the sides of the bowl as needed.

Combine the remaining 3 cups flour, the baking powder, and salt in a medium bowl. With the mixer on low speed, gradually beat the flour mixture into the egg mixture, alternating with the evaporated milk and the orange juice. Fold in the orange rind. Pour the batter into the bundt pan and bake until a toothpick inserted into the center comes out clean, 70 to 80 minutes. Cool in the pan for 20 minutes. Invert the cake onto a large plate and lift off the bundt pan.

C I T R U S S O A K : Whisk the confectioners' sugar, orange juice and lemon juice in a small bowl until the sugar dissolves. While the cake is still warm, pierce it all over with a skewer. Brush the glaze over the cake with a pastry brush until it is completely absorbed. Cut into slices and serve.

Instant Lemon Pudding Cake

SERVES 12 TO 16

This cake is one of David's favorite desserts from childhood, especially the lemon glaze.

CAKE

8	tablespoons (1 stick) plus 1 tablespoon unsalted butter, at room temperature
2	cups plus 2 tablespoons all-purpose flour
1½	cups sugar
4	large eggs, lightly beaten
1	cup skim milk
1	3.4-ounce package instant lemon pudding
¼	cup canola oil
3½	teaspoons baking powder
2	teaspoons finely grated lemon rind
1½	teaspoons lemon extract
1	teaspoon vanilla extract
1	teaspoon salt

GLAZE

2	cups confectioners' sugar
¼	cup fresh lemon juice

Preheat the oven to 350 degrees F. Butter and flour a 12-cup bundt pan, using 1 tablespoon of the butter and 2 tablespoons of the flour.

CAKE: Beat the sugar and eggs with an electric mixer on medium speed in a large bowl for 30 seconds. Add the remaining 2 cups flour, the remaining 8 tablespoons butter, the milk, pudding mix, oil, baking powder, lemon rind, lemon extract, vanilla, and salt. Beat on high speed for 3 minutes, scraping the bowl as needed. Pour the batter into the bundt pan and bake for 40 to 45 minutes, or until a toothpick inserted into the center comes out clean. Cool for 20 minutes. Invert the cake onto a large plate and lift off the bundt pan.

GLAZE: Whisk the confectioners' sugar and lemon juice in a medium bowl until smooth and creamy. When the cake is cool, drizzle the glaze over the cake. Cut into slices and serve.

Angel Food–
Strawberry Delight

SERVES 12

This is a very light, fat-free dessert.
You can substitute other berries or peaches for the strawberries,
depending on what's in season.

CAKE

1   cup sifted cake flour
1½   cups sugar
1½   cups large egg whites (from 10–12 large eggs)
1½   teaspoons cream of tartar
¼   teaspoon salt
1½   teaspoons vanilla extract

TOPPING

3   large egg whites
6   tablespoons superfine sugar
½   teaspoon vanilla extract
1   pint strawberries, hulled, each cut into 3–4 slices

CAKE: Preheat the oven to 350 degrees F.

Combine the flour and ¾ cup of the sugar in a large bowl. Beat the egg whites, cream of tartar, and salt with an electric mixer on high speed in a separate large bowl until fluffy. Add the remaining ¾ cup of sugar to the egg whites, 2 tablespoons at a time, beating well after each addition. Beat until stiff peaks form, then beat in the vanilla.

Sift the dry ingredients over the egg whites, about 2 tablespoons at a time, gently folding after each addition.

Pour the batter into an ungreased 10-inch tube pan and cut through the batter gently with a knife to remove any large air bubbles. Bake for 40 to 50 minutes, or until the cake is golden brown with dry cracks on top. Remove from the oven and invert the pan on an upside-down funnel immediately. Cool for 1 hour before removing the cake from the pan.

TOPPING: Beat the egg whites with an electric mixer on high speed in a large bowl until fluffy. Add the sugar, 1 tablespoon at a time, beating well after each addition. Beat until the egg whites are stiff and glossy, then beat in the vanilla.

Preheat the broiler.

Remove the cake from the pan by running a spatula around the edges and inverting it on an ovenproof serving platter. Lift off the pan. Top with the egg-white mixture. Place under the broiler 4 inches from the heat source and broil until the topping is golden, 2 to 3 minutes, watching carefully so it doesn't burn. Top with the strawberries and serve.

Banana Cake

SERVES 8 TO 10

No one will notice the absence of the usual sour cream
and nuts in this rich cake. The amount of banana per serving is
headache-safe, as long as you don't overindulge.

8   tablespoons (1 stick) plus 1 tablespoon unsalted
     butter for greasing the pan
1½ cups all-purpose flour
1   cup sugar
¼   cup skim milk
1   large egg
1   teaspoon baking powder
1   teaspoon baking soda
1   teaspoon vanilla extract
2–3 very ripe bananas, mashed (about 2½ cups)

Preheat the oven to 350 degrees F. Butter a 9-x-5-x-3-inch loaf
pan, using the 1 tablespoon butter.

Combine the flour, sugar, the remaining 8 tablespoons butter, the
milk, egg, baking powder, baking soda, and vanilla in a large bowl and
stir until smooth. Fold the bananas into the batter. Spoon the batter
into the loaf pan and bake for 45 minutes, or until a toothpick inserted into the center comes out clean. Cool in the pan on a rack. Run a
knife around the edges of the pan, invert the cake over a plate, and lift
off the pan. Slice and serve.

Raspberry Soufflés

SERVES 6

Festive enough for the most elegant dinner party, these soufflés
are low in calories and fat-free.

1   tablespoon unsalted butter
1   tablespoon sugar
1   10-ounce package frozen raspberries in syrup,
     thawed
4   large egg whites
½   cup superfine sugar

Preheat the oven to 375 degrees F. Butter 6 individual soufflé
dishes, using the 1 tablespoon butter, and lightly coat them with the 1
tablespoon sugar.

Place the raspberries in a food processor and process until smooth.

Beat the egg whites with an electric mixer in a large bowl until soft
peaks form. Beat in the superfine sugar, 1 tablespoon at a time, until
the egg whites are stiff and glossy. Fold in the raspberry puree.

Spoon the raspberry mixture into the soufflé dishes. Bake for 12 to
15 minutes, or until the soufflés are puffed and lightly golden. Serve
immediately.

Glazed Pear Tarts

SERVES 6

Excellent frozen puff pastry is available in the freezer case
of the supermarket. If you keep some on hand, you can whip up
impressive last-minute desserts like these tarts.

POACHED PEARS

6 ripe pears
4 cups water
1½ cups sugar
Juice of 2 medium lemons, strained
Rind of 2 medium lemons, cut in
½-inch-wide strips
2 tablespoons vanilla extract

GLAZE

¾ cup apricot jam

PASTRY

½ 17.3-ounce package frozen puff-pastry dough
1 large egg
1 teaspoon water

POACHED PEARS: Peel the pears, leaving their stems on.
Cut a small slice from the bottom of each pear so they will stand
upright.

Combine the water, sugar, lemon juice, lemon rind, and vanilla in
a medium saucepan over medium-low heat. Bring to a simmer and add
the pears. Adjust the heat to keep the syrup just below a simmer, and
cook, uncovered, for 12 to 15 minutes, or until the pears are tender.
Let cool in the syrup.

GLAZE: Transfer 1 cup of the syrup to a small saucepan over medium-high heat and add the apricot jam. Bring to a boil and boil, stirring, for 3 to 4 minutes, or until thickened.

PASTRY: Preheat the oven to 450 degrees F.

Roll out the pastry sheet into an 8-x-10-inch rectangle. Cut it in half lengthwise, then cut each half into thirds, forming a total of 6 rectangles. Place the pastry rectangles on a moistened baking sheet.

Beat the egg and the water in a small bowl. Brush the tops of the pastry rectangles with the egg mixture. Using a sharp knife, cut lightly into the pastry in a crosshatch design.

Bake until puffed, brown, and crisp, about 15 minutes. When the pastry is cool enough to handle, split the rectangles, separating the top layers from the bottom layers.

Spoon the glaze over the pears. Place a pool of about 1½ tablespoons glaze on each of 6 plates. Place the bottom of a puff-pastry rectangle on each plate, top with a glazed pear, then top with the top half of the puff-pastry rectangle, setting it on an angle. Serve immediately.

Grape Tarts
with Vanilla Pastry Cream

SERVES 6

These tarts look like a fancy restaurant dessert.
The tangy grapes contrast well with the smooth pastry cream,
creating a unique and satisfying dessert.

CRUST

12 ounces (about 1 box) vanilla wafers
2 tablespoons unsalted butter, melted

PASTRY CREAM

6 large egg yolks
½ cup sugar
Pinch salt
½ cup all-purpose flour
1¾ cups skim milk, heated
1 tablespoon vanilla extract

GLAZE

1 cup apricot preserves
3 tablespoons sugar
1 tablespoon fresh lemon juice

1½ cups seedless red grapes, stemmed
and halved lengthwise
1½ cups seedless purple grapes, stemmed
and halved lengthwise

CRUST: Chop the vanilla wafers into fine crumbs in a food processor. Transfer the crumbs to a small bowl and stir in the butter. Line 6 removable-bottom 3-to-4-inch tart pans with the wafer mixture. Chill in the refrigerator.

PASTRY CREAM: Whisk the egg yolks in a medium saucepan, gradually adding the sugar and salt. Whisk until the yolk mixture is thick and lemon colored. Sift the flour over the egg mixture and whisk it in. Gradually whisk in the milk.

Bring to a boil over medium heat, whisking constantly. The custard will start to get lumpy but will become smooth as you whisk. Reduce the heat to low and stir with a wooden spoon. Cook for 2 minutes more, stirring. Press the sauce through a fine strainer into a medium bowl and stir in vanilla. Cover the surface of the pastry cream with plastic wrap and refrigerate.

GLAZE: Heat the apricot preserves, sugar, and lemon juice in a small saucepan over medium heat, stirring, until the sugar dissolves. Press the preserves through a fine strainer into a small bowl, then return to the saucepan and keep warm over low heat.

Fill the tart shells with the pastry cream. Cover the top with the grape halves cut side down, alternating red and purple, arranged close together in a circular pattern. Brush the grapes lightly with the glaze. Chill the tarts in the refrigerator. Remove the outer ring from the tart pans and let come to room temperature before serving.

Orange Soufflés in Oranges

MAKES 6 SOUFFLÉS

These individual soufflés are more stable than one large one,
so there is less danger of that bugaboo, the collapsing soufflé.
The soufflé is spooned into hollowed-out oranges,
which make colorful substitutes for soufflé dishes.

  6 **sugar cubes**
  7 **very large navel oranges**
  2 **teaspoons orange juice**
  3 **tablespoons unsalted butter**
  3 **tablespoons all-purpose flour**
  ¾ **cup 1% milk, heated**
  3 **large eggs, separated**
  6 **tablespoons sugar**
  ¼ **teaspoon cream of tartar**
1½ **teaspoons orange extract**
  ½ **teaspoon vanilla extract**

Preheat the oven to 450 degrees F.

Rub all 6 sugar cubes all over the skin of 1 of the oranges to coat
the cubes with the zest, oil, and color of the orange. Place the zest-cov-
ered sugar cubes in a small bowl with the orange juice.

Cut a ¾-inch slice from the navel ends of the remaining 6 oranges.
Scoop out the insides of the oranges, leaving the skins intact. Cut a
very thin slice off the stem end of the oranges so they will stand
upright. Place the oranges on a cookie sheet.

Melt the butter in a small saucepan over low heat. Stir in the flour and whisk until smooth. Add the milk and whisk constantly until the sauce is thickened and smooth. Remove from the heat and add the egg yolks, whisking constantly. Return to the heat, bring to a boil, and boil, whisking, for 10 seconds. Remove from the heat and stir in the sugar and the sugar-cube mixture, beating well until they are incorporated. Cool for 20 minutes.

Meanwhile, bake the orange skins for 5 minutes, or until dried out. Remove from the oven.

Beat the egg whites and cream of tartar with an electric mixer in a large bowl until stiff. Stir in the orange extract and vanilla. Stir half of the egg whites into the yolk mixture to lighten it, then fold in the rest of the egg whites.

Spoon the soufflé into the orange skins, filling them three-fourths full. Bake for 15 minutes, or until the soufflés are puffed and brown and a toothpick inserted into the center comes out clean. Serve immediately.

Index

About the Authors

—— ❧ ——

David R. Marks, M.D., is medical director of the New England Center for Headache in Stamford, Connecticut. He is a health reporter for WVIT-TV, an NBC station in Hartford. Laura Marks, M.D., is a pediatrician. They live in Westport, Connecticut.